KINGDOM

NUTRITION

KINGDOM KIDS NUTRITION

A Journey to Emotional and Behavioral Health

KELLI SCHULTE

Published by XP Publishing
A department of Christian Services Association
P.O. Box 1017, Maricopa, Arizona 85139
www.XPpublishing.com

ISBN: 978-1-936101-64-1

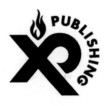

Printed in the United States of America. For Worldwide Distribution.

DEDICATIONS

I thank my Lord and Savior, *Jesus Christ*, who inspires my careful selection and preparation of the food we eat. Through this revelation, He has brought health, healing and life to my family and others. I praise the Lord every day for blessing our family.

I adore my daughter *Hannah*, who blesses my life and is the driving force behind our journey into natural health. Thank you for teaching me and forgiving me when I make mistakes. Most of all, thank you for loving me and putting up with all my experimental cooking!

To *Paul, Lilli, Matthew,* and *Michael* for your patience through all the recipes, diets, and changes along this journey. Thank you for allowing me to follow God's call on my life to bring optimal health to others. I love you so much!

To *Robin Flis*, my mentor, friend and prayer warrior on this exciting pilgrimage. Your hours of prayer, consultation, and dedication to my family and me help make all this possible. Thank you, Robin, for allowing God to use you to assist us in growing in the knowledge of the power of prayer, natural health, and healing foods.

To *Carol Martinez* and *Michelle Burkett*, who came along side of me, putting in hours of editing, formatting, and making it possible for this book to become a reality! A special thank you to both of you!

And finally, I honor the *Moms* who are dedicated to bringing health, nutrition and healing to their families through a healthy, nutritious, and tasty diet!

CONTENTS

FOREWORD

It was the third week of classes and Hannah wanted me to walk her in to school. Because we strolled in about ten minutes early, we sat in the hallway for a moment, where Hannah recognized one of her new friends; she turned to me and said, "I think I'll go to class now." I watched as she walked away from me with a spring to her step and such confidence that it brought tears of joy to my eyes. She approached her friend and began talking, smiling, and laughing — she was having fun!

As I walked out of South Heights Christian Classes that morning, (the school Hannah attends once a week), I could taste victory! It was a sunny and cool, crisp fall morning in Minnesota; I closed my eyes, took a deep breath and soaked in the moment. My whole being was filled with joy and excitement for what lay ahead for my daughter — a life filled with joy and promise.

Hannah, who will be 13 in December, walks in freedom! Her passions are dance and the visual arts and she spends many hours every week in ballet, point ballet and jazz dance classes, as well as other classes that develop her artistic gifts. She also loves developing computer websites and blogs and is very active, serving along side my husband in children's ministry! Hannah is a gifted, confident, and creative young lady, who is surrounded by friends filled with hopes and dreams for the future.

But is wasn't always that way...

INTRODUCTION

The Lord is near to the brokenhearted
and saves those who are crushed in spirit.

Psalm 34:18

I entered the pediatrician's office literally dragging my scream-ing three-year old, Hannah, through the door. I was absolutely frazzled. Hannah was clutching my leg and my brand new baby girl, Lilli, was also screaming as I carried her in the car seat. Sweat dripping down my forehead. I thought maybe I should just join in with them and break down bawling right there in the doctor's lobby. But, attempting to be a "good" mom, I tried to ignore my two screaming children, tuck my desperation and frustration deep down inside, and politely check them in.

The nurse, sensing my distress, immediately stepped in. She grabbed the baby and rushed us back into a room. When she took the baby, I was free to sweep up my other screaming daughter, her arms and legs flailing, and follow the nurse. As soon as we got to the room, the nurse handed my baby back to me and left. I had to stand against the door to keep Hannah inside. The baby continued to scream, so I tried to rock her while using all my body weight to hold the door shut and keep my three-year-old from escaping. Exasperated, I anxiously waited for the doctor to arrive. I thought, "Wow, that was an ugly scene, but now he will finally know what I've been trying to get him to understand for almost three years." Time after time I had told him, "My daughter gets so upset and out of control that she cannot get herself to calm down," but neither he nor the office staff seemed to "get it." However, today in the midst of such chaos I felt some hope. At *last* they would see and give me some answers!

At this point my daughter Hannah was having these massive meltdowns for hours on end, multiple times per day. I had tried to explain to doctors how intense these times were but it always seemed to fall on deaf ears. I was actually excited that today the nurses had seen her outburst for the first time (and what turned out to be the last). "Finally, they will really believe and help me," I thought.

As we waited and waited for the doctor, my daughter eventually calmed down. When he entered the room she was sitting with me reading a book. "You had a bit of a time getting in here I heard." I just smiled. He then said, "Well, some days are just like that." He didn't understand that *every* day was like this!

Once again, my hopeful expectations regarding the doctors went unfulfilled. They simply didn't get it. The whole experience was chalked up to "jealousy" of the new baby. I left feeling defeated and alone. I knew my daughter was struggling and hurting. I loved her so much, but nothing I did helped her.

This scene had been playing over and over since my daughter was ten months old. She seemed so sensitive to everything, and her responses were so extreme!

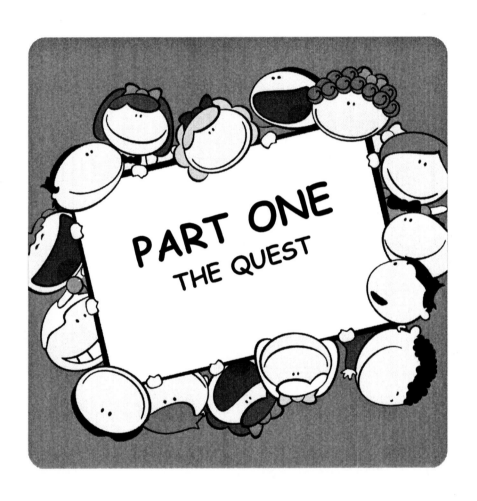

PART ONE
THE QUEST

From Hannah's Heart:

Life for our family wasn't always easy – it had a lot of twists and turns. But it has taught us a very important lesson on perseverance, how to push through hard obstacles and come out of them stronger than we went into them! I hope that through my family's story you find hope and courage.

God bless each and every one of you who have read this book and taken steps into your own personal battleground that God has set up for you to conquer. Stay strong and trust God, because He LOVES YOU more than you can imagine!

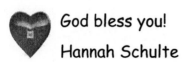 God bless you!
Hannah Schulte

Chapter 1

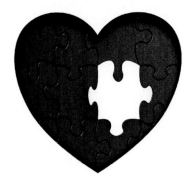

THE WAY IT WAS

As I look back upon my life before I had my own children, I can see God's hand preparing me for them. I worked successfully for nine years with special needs kids, never realizing that God had me in a "boot camp" of sorts in preparation for my own daughter. He gave me tools and training in how to deal with all types of behaviors. He provided me with a firm foundation of health and nutrition to build upon, and He built my resolve and passion to fight for my daughter as I had fought for so many students before her.

HANNAH

On December 18, 1998, my life was changed forever as I looked into the big, alert, wide-open eyes of my new baby daughter, Hannah Ruth. I knew she was very special. Looking at her, I knew without a doubt that there must be a God. This was all too incredible for words. Love for her went deep into my soul; there was nothing I wouldn't do for her.

Everything with Hannah was great until she was about ten months old. She caught a cold at the beginning of October, and by the end of the month she had not yet recovered. I took her to the doctor, who said that Hannah would need to have a nebulizer treatment because her airways were very swollen and she was wheezing slightly.

Little did I know that this was the beginning of a three-year bout with asthma, numerous respiratory infections, many trips to the ER in the middle of the night, and hours of nebulizer treatments. By December, we were doing up to twelve of these treatments per day to keep her breathing under control. She also started developing chronic ear infections requiring multiple rounds of antibiotics. And strep throat became a problem that led to more antibiotics. At age three, the doctor put her on a daily dose of Singulair to control her asthma. She slowly began to grow out of it and things decreased in intensity. Thankfully, by four-and-a-half she was totally off her nebulizer.

TANTRUMS AND MELTDOWNS

As we were dealing with all the respiratory issues, we were also going through the "let-her-cry-it-out" phase. As a small baby, Hannah had always been the easiest child to put to bed – I would just lay her down and she would go to sleep. But then at ten months, she would stand in her crib, shake the bars and jump up and down while crying hysterically. I consulted the pediatrician, sharing that bedtime was getting worse, to the point that even going into her room made her cry. As an infant, she had never really napped for more than an hour but she had gone to bed like clockwork, waking up at 10pm, 2am and 6am nightly. Now she was screaming when we put her to bed.

The doctor chalked it up to Hannah being "strong-willed" and told me that she just needed to learn who was boss. He advised me to let her "cry it out." The first night, Hannah cried three hours and 45 minutes. The nights following continued to be just as bad. Letting her cry it out simply didn't work.

Then the doctor changed his tune and said that she was having early separation anxiety. He gave us another plan: we were to put Hannah in her bed, wait five minutes, go in and comfort her, put her back in bed, and leave the room. We were to repeat this sequence, extending the time before going back in the room, by five-minute increments. We did this for hours each night, trying to make it work – but it didn't. We ended up just cuddling her until she fell asleep. We did what we could and somehow made it through those long, sleepless nights.

STRONG-WILLED?

In other areas of development, my daughter was excelling at an incredible pace. At 18 months she was talking fluently in full sentences. She was fun, curious, and fully potty trained.

However, at that age I noticed that one of her eyes would cross occasionally. We took her to a pediatric eye specialist and found that Hannah had one eye stronger than the other. So, she wore glasses and we did a regiment of patching the strong eye to make the other eye work harder and get stronger. We did this for about two years. We always allowed her to pick her own eyeglasses. She has had a sense of fashion since the day she was born. She always looked so cute!

But the tantrums and meltdowns continued, until Hannah had the reputation within the family as the "strong-willed child." I read the book, *The Strong-Willed Child* by Dr. James Dobson, and she fit the description perfectly. I even went to one of their parenting seminars. Though the seminar encouraged me, there was a problem: none of the strategies mentioned in the book worked for my daughter. It seemed the more we spoke about how strong-willed she was, the worse things became.

I repeatedly spoke with the pediatrician about Hannah's determined behavior and meltdowns that could last for *hours*. He told me to put her in her room and leave her there. So, I did. I would leave her, by herself, in her room. She would kick, scream, yell, hit, and come running out again. I would return her to her room, over and over throughout the day, with no success. The pediatrician suggested

I put a lock on the outside of the door so she couldn't come out. So we did, but she would just kick, scream, and hit the door for hours. She became so frantic – we could tell this was only scaring her.

We talked to her pediatrician again and he gave more suggestions. None of them worked. When she got upset, there was nothing that would help. The pediatrician continued to tell me that everything she was doing was "normal" and there was nothing to worry about, but in my heart I knew something was desperately wrong.

We went about life the best we could, stumbling along in frustration, watching our daughter grow, her behavior becoming more and more erratic and aggressive. I had learned many tools in my years of teaching, but I had run out of answers for my Hannah. Life was slowly spinning out of control.

GLIMPSES OF LIGHT

Things went on without much improvement for the next year. However, when she was two and a half, Hannah was very excited when I became pregnant with our second daughter, Lilli. She wanted a sister and told me that God told her she would have one. I kept trying to caution her that it might be a boy but she was adamant that it was a sister. She even went so far as to tell me that if it was a boy she was not going to love it. My husband and I decided we better get an ultrasound to find out, so we could prepare her if indeed it was a boy.

We walked into the doctor's office for the ultrasound with Hannah in tow. As everything was being hooked up, Hannah kept asking, "Where is my baby sister?" I kept saying, "It might be a boy. Let's see." After a while, the technician said, "You're right, it is definitely a baby sister." "See mommy, I was right. I am going to have a baby sister." I was shocked. This was one of the first times we saw God speak to and through Hannah. As this began to occur with frequency, we just thought, "Wow, church is doing its job – our daughter already knows who God is, at age three."

Not long after that, we were at a wedding, and during the service Hannah said, "Mommy, Jesus is here."

"Where?" I asked.

"Sitting right up there," she said, pointing to the left side of the cross. "Above the couple being married."

I asked, "What does He look like?"

She replied, "He's older, with blue hair and a beard. He is smiling."

I half-heartedly believed her, but the other part of me didn't know, though I sure thought it was cute!

NEW HOME – NEW ISSUES

When Hannah was four, we moved into another home. I had been working part time and driving a half-hour each way to work with both girls. We decided to buy a bigger home closer to my work so we wouldn't spend so much time in the car. We found a house two miles from the school where I was teaching. It was a quiet neighborhood with a wooded lot where the kids could play. The move went well, although it was hard on Hannah. We were finding that change and transition, even on a small scale, were not her strengths.

In the new home new issues boiled up to the surface. She became obsessed about washing her hands even when they weren't dirty. She refused to go in our new basement because she was fearful. For five years she never went into the basement alone. Not even to watch television.

Hannah became fearful in other places, too. She would become visibly frightened in a store or someone's home and say, "I gotta go, I gotta go!" We just thought it was more erratic behavior coming out. We later learned that Hannah was actually sensing things that many others don't see or feel, and it was scaring her.

A DANGEROUS TURN

For several years things continued along in the same way, but Hannah's behavior escalated when she entered Kindergarten at age five. On one occasion, when she was invited to a birthday party, we went to the local toy store to get a gift for her friend. Our family rule is that when we go shopping for a gift, we don't shop for anything else, so our focus is on what will bless our friend. She knew this family agreement and had never struggled with it in the past. We walked into the store and something caught Hannah's eye. I reminded her that we were there for her friend's birthday gift and we were not going to look at anything for ourselves. She didn't like that answer and began to cry and yell. I picked her up and dragged her out of the store, flailing, kicking, screaming, and crying. Beads of sweat dripped off my brow, but she needed to learn. I put her in the back seat of the car, buckled her in, and went to the front seat.

As I pulled out of the parking lot and began driving down the frontage road, my daughter unbuckled her belt, crawled between the front seats and grabbed the steering wheel, yelling, "Go back, Mommy, go back!" I said, "No, we're going home. That's not the way we act in a store." She refused to sit down or buckle up. I got out my cell phone, dialed 911 and put my finger on the green button. I told Hannah it was against the law for her to not be in her seat belt and I would need to call the police to buckle her in, if she would not do it herself. She quickly sat down and put on her seat belt. I drove home with my finger on the green button, to keep her in it. In the half-hour drive home, she took everything she could find out of the back seat of the car and threw it at me: water bottle, ice scraper, clothes, etc. When we finally arrived at the house, I put Hannah in her room to calm down. My husband then took over and sat outside her door.

That day both of my daughters also had dental appointments. Hannah loved her dentist, but after my harrowing experience in the car I wasn't up to taking her out again. I told her that as a consequence for her behavior she would have to stay home. It was not a surprise that Hannah resumed her tantrum. I left with my younger daughter Lilli and we drove to the dentist where she refused to open her mouth – what a day! Arriving back at the house, I could hear Hannah still blowing a total fit.

When I walked into her room, she ran and clung to me, melting into a puddle of remorse. This happened every time. She would get so upset and then it was as if her neurological system would break down, she'd fall into a puddle and sob, saying, "I'm sorry, I'm sorry."

MEDICATION

When she finally relaxed, I took my husband aside and said, "That's it. I'm not doing this anymore. She's going on medication to-morrow. We can't continue to live this way." We didn't know what else to do. As teachers, we were trained that if a child has a chemical imbalance and you give them the drug that balances out the chemicals – everything is fine. It made sense to my husband and me, so I made the appointment.

The next day we went to a new pediatrician who sent us to a behavior specialist to discuss medication, a child psychologist for an evaluation, and a physical therapist for her tippy-toe walking.

I began with the behavior specialist that afternoon. I went through Hannah's health history and described the behavior issues we were having. He quickly diagnosed her as having anxiety with obsessive-compulsive tendencies. He put her on 10 mg of Lexapro.

I went directly to the pharmacy, picked up the medication and we started the meds that day. It made me sick, but I did not know what else to do at the time. I was on anti-anxiety medication and had been for years, so half of me thought, "Well, she's my daughter – of course she needs medication." My husband and I prayed that God would make it very clear that we had done the right thing. The next morning

Hannah woke up and soon we heard her singing away in the shower. That was incredible! She was happy and bubbly all day long. Our prayer was answered – we were at peace with our decision. Little did we know that the medication was only to be a temporary fix – a "band aid" – until we had the revelation of what would bring Hannah true healing. God used medication to bring a brief moment of peace in our journey. But at the same time, the next season of living in therapy and doctors' offices was birthed!

Chapter 2

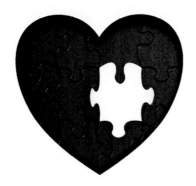

DOCTORS, DOCTORS, DOCTORS

O ur life became a traveling road show from one doctor to the
next. I now had three children, and everywhere I went there
was a trail of little ones following me like ducklings from car
to office and back again.

At this time, we had to deal with another challenge that had nothing to do with her behavior and emotional issues. While we thought
that our daughter was strong-willed and extremely sensitive, we also
believed that she was gifted, because she just skipped crawling and
began walking at ten months. We were unaware that this was a red
flag. Then, shortly after she learned to walk, she began to "tippy-toe"
walk, another missed warning sign. And, when I had spoken to the
doctor about this at her two year check up, he had said it was it was
totally normal and nothing to worry about.

Now we know that tippy-toe walking is a sure sign of a sensory
issue, if they do not grow out of it by age three. The reason she was

always on her tippy-toes is that she didn't like how things felt on her feet. We just thought someday she would be a ballerina.

But now, several years later, we were facing a harsh reality. The physical therapist found that Hannah's Achilles tendons and hamstrings were extremely tight due to her tippy-toe walking. He explained that they would have to do casting to stretch out her tendons and apply leg immobilizers (knee braces) to stretch out her hamstrings. Our five-year-old daughter ended up with casts on both legs, from her feet to her knees, and at bedtime she had braces on both of her legs that went from her hip to her cast. This kept her knees in constant stretch, causing the tendons to gain flexibility.

This was a three-month process. Each week they would remove the cast, stretch her leg a little more and recast it to hold the stretch. Keeping the braces on her knees at night was impossible. The doctor told us that if Hannah did not keep her braces on at night for one full week, she would need to get Botox injections at her next appointment to relax the muscles and get them to begin stretching.

We left the appointment terrified about the potential of injecting our daughter with botulism. We were determined to keep those braces on, no matter the cost. That first night was the battle of the braces. We gave Hannah Motrin in an attempt to reduce the pain. After about twenty minutes, we put the braces on her and tucked her in bed. In moments, she began to scream, "It hurts, it hurts! Please, Mom, stop! Take them off!" My husband and I stood firm as she screamed and screamed. I finally reached my breaking point and had to leave the room.

A Miracle

I went to my bedroom and cried out to God, praying that God would heal Hannah's legs and that she would not need the injections. I felt a peace fall over me – I knew Hannah's legs were going to be fine. All my fear and anxiety disappeared and faith entered my heart – I knew God was going to heal her legs. I walked back into Hannah's room where my husband was in full-on battle with our daughter. I said, "If God is going to heal her, He can heal her without the braces." My husband was in agreement, so we took off the braces.

I had begun reaching out to God, but only in times of crisis such as this one. In the midst of these cries of desperation He showed me He was really there and that He truly loved my daughter.

A week later, we walked into the physical therapist's office, where the doctor took off the casts and measured Hannah's range of motion. He did it once, then again. He looked at our daughter and said, "Wow, you must have done an awesome job wearing your braces this week. I have never seen such a gain in range of motion. Your foot went from a minus-two to plus-twelve." He looked at us and said, "This is unheard of – way to go, guys!"

Hannah told the doctor, "I never wore my braces. I just prayed to God all the way here that I would not need to get the shots." We confirmed that she never wore the braces but that God had healed her. The doctor never commented; he was just silent. This was the first physical work of God we had ever seen in our lives. He had answered our prayers and we were on our way to adding daily prayer to our regimen of getting our daughter "figured out."

She did continue using the casts for three months. After the casting, she wore braces from the knee down for about a year, followed by in-shoe braces. It was a long journey, but all of this was successful in getting her tendons to stretch; she now walks normally.

Hits and Misses

We began weekly visits to a psychologist who gave us many suggestions that would prove to be ineffective. When Hannah got upset, it was as if she was "gone." We would look at her but she was somewhere else in her head, and we couldn't get her back until she crashed into a puddle of tears and remorse. My heart would break for her every time.

Once she began taking medication, all was well for a while. Hannah was having fewer meltdowns, seemed a bit happier and more agreeable. Then slowly, things began to go downhill again. Concerned that the medication was no longer working, I went back to the behavior specialist who had prescribed it, and he increased her dosage. Now my six-year-old was on an adult dose of 20 mg of Lexapro. Again, we saw marked improvement for a few months.

At the end of Hannah's first-grade year, we switched to a Christian psychologist. Her specialty was childhood anxiety and sensory processing disorders. Hannah really liked her. She diagnosed Hannah with anxiety, depression, and obsessive-compulsive disorder (OCD). She also identified "Mr. Worry" for Hannah. She told her that Mr. Worry tries to get us to believe lies so that we will do what he wants instead of what we want to do. This was very interesting because Hannah had been saying that voices were telling her to do the wrong thing. Even though she knew it was wrong, the voices were stronger than her ability to stand against them.

TOOLS FOR HANNAH

During this time, I began attending a Bible study where we were learning about spiritual warfare. I realized that my daughter was under attack from the enemy and the voices in her mind were not from God. With the help of the psychologist, who taught Hannah that she was in control of Mr. Worry and Mr. Worry was not in charge of her, Hannah slowly began to take back control. This took a long time. It wasn't until Hannah was in third grade and receiving sound teaching at our church that she really took hold of the authority she had over the enemy. She learned that the negative thoughts, words and voices she heard had no place in her, and because Jesus lives in her she had *His* power. She could actually say, "No" to the negative thoughts and voices – then speak the truth (what God would say). For example, she often thought, "Your mom doesn't love you." When she would have that thought or hear that being whispered in her ear, she would now say, "No, my mom loves me!"

We began writing down and tracking these lies and having her speak the truth out loud daily. As we continued to grow and worked more with the Christian psychologist, spiritual connections began to surface. I saw that what was going on with Hannah was more than behavior; it was also a spiritual journey. At first, it all sounded pretty crazy to me. I was raised Catholic and never thought there was a spiritual aspect to our world. I just figured the reason to go to church was so I could go to heaven – it didn't have much to do with daily life. But now, spiritual reality was staring me in the face, as I was living it with my daughter. The question was: what do I do? The answer continued to unravel over the next years.

At this time we were going to a physical therapist and psychologist every week and Hannah was taking 20 mg of Lexapro daily. We thought we had finally found the "cure" to bring relief to her and peace to our family. But within a month of her dose increase, things again began to deteriorate. As the meds wore off, the behaviors and meltdowns came back even more intensely! We were at our wits' end and I was once again at my breaking point. I cried out to God to help my daughter and reveal a path that would bring healing to her. I knew life could not go on like this. Hannah was becoming stronger, smarter and more violent with each day.

During this time I was given the name of a Christian pediatrician. We prayed about it and made an appointment. I was exasperated as I walked into her office. "How can I help you?" she asked.

I answered, "God sent me to you to heal my daughter."

She laughed and said, "OK then, tell me about your daughter." She ordered a full blood work-up and tested for every possible allergy. She had us continue to see our Christian psychologist and have an occupational therapy assessment with another Christian practitioner. We didn't see it at the time, but God's hand was at work. Except for the physical therapist, the entire team working with our daughter was now Christian. They were not only treating her physically and mentally but they were praying for her as well.

Help Me, Mommy!

A typical week included multiple visits both in and out of the city to see the occupational therapist (in Edina, 25 minutes away), physical therapist (Minnetonka, 20 minutes away) and psychologist (downtown Minneapolis, 45 minutes away). Our life consisted of doctors' offices, the car, and occasionally I would get her to school. With all these doctors, nothing had really changed. I returned to our pediatrician because we needed something else. What we were doing was not working.

One morning, Hannah was getting dressed and could not find anything to wear that "felt right." Everything was either too loose or too tight and all the tags and seams itched. She began frantically running around. This had been an increasing problem – Hannah would meltdown in the morning and it would take me until noon to calm her and get her to school.

The school was not happy with this and didn't believe anything I had to say, as Hannah was the perfect child in school. They said it was my anxiety that was plaguing her, "toughen up" and if needed, bring her to school in her pajamas so she knew who was boss. This particular morning I decided to follow their advice. I asked Hannah to get dressed so we could get to school. When I walked in her room, she was in her underwear, running around in circles with her long blonde hair all ratted in knots, going every which way. I said, "I'm going to get your brother and sister in the car and then I will get you. Dressed or not, I am taking you to school right now."

She yelled, "No, Mommy, no!"

When I came back from putting the other two kids in the van, Hannah was still not dressed. She was huddled in the corner of her bed clutching her knees, head buried. As I looked at her, my heart broke. She looked like a terrified, caged animal as she sat there crying. When I handed her some clothes, she looked at me with a vacant look and said, "Get away from me." I picked her up still undressed and she began flailing and screaming. I carried her to the car with her scream-ing, "Help me, help me, Mommy!"

This was the problem – every time she would get upset she would yell, "Help me, help me," and everything I did made it worse. I placed her in the van, handed her clothes to her, and shut the door. My gut was saying that this was so wrong! But, "they" said I had to get her to school. Hannah continued to scream as we pulled out of the driveway. Then while I drove, Hannah scurried to the front of the van and grabbed the steering wheel, causing us to swerve across the road! I just reacted by pushing her into the back of the van. I rapidly pulled over to the side of the road and looked back to see my little five-year-old daughter in a bundle on the floor, now petrified of me. I reached for her and she said, "No, get away! Get away, you're scary!"

As calmly as I could, I responded, "Hannah, what you did could have killed us if another car had been coming. It is very serious. Mommy just reacted to get you away from the steering wheel. I'm sorry."

I turned to face the road. The car was silent. There was no way I could take her to school in this condition. The days of listening to all the advice from the world was over. I began to listen to my heart, the still small voice of God. At that time I didn't know that's what it was. I just knew that when I followed that voice, things went much better. The days of listening to all the advice from the "world" was over; I was going to do what I thought was best for my daughter.

I was able to make an immediate appointment for Hannah with the occupational therapist and dropped off my other children at a friend's house to avoid having them sit through another therapy session. I was so beyond tears – I could feel a hardening of my heart. I just couldn't take any more. Hannah was much calmer after her session with the therapist and once again, I delivered her to school at 11:30am.

A few days later, Hannah was throwing a fit in her bedroom and then came out and asked me where my knitting needles were. When I asked why, she answered, "I want to stab myself with them." She was six years old! Where was this coming from? Why was this all happening despite the medication? I calmly answered, "No, you can't use my knitting needles to stab yourself." I basically just ignored her, thinking she was looking for attention. Suddenly, my daughter Lilli came in and said, "Mommy, the kitty is biting Hannah." Hannah had gotten the cat and was squeezing him so he would bite her. I told her to let the cat go and she said, "No, it feels good." I rescued the cat and called my husband at work. We decided to document with video what was going on, because it seemed no one believed how severe all of this was.

The next week, my husband and I took a video of one of Hannah's meltdowns and showed it to her occupational therapist. The staff had a hard time believing any of this with Hannah, because she was a "perfect" patient. That was part of the problem. She was "perfect" everywhere outside of the home and then when she got home, she would meltdown. Hannah would say that she couldn't be herself when she was away from home.

When I showed the occupational therapy team the video, they finally were able to see the vacant, empty look Hannah usually got during these meltdowns. Their response was, "Hannah needs to have a neuro-psych evaluation as soon as possible!"

A LABEL?

We were sent to a testing center that diagnoses and treats children on the autism spectrum. We spent one full day having Hannah evaluated by numerous doctors, psychologists and social workers. I was actually hoping and praying that this team of doctors would diagnose Hannah with autism, or some form of autism spectrum disorder, so I could get support from the school instead of the condemnation I was currently experiencing. Everything I read that had impacted my daughter was about autistic children. I knew without a doubt that she was on the autism spectrum! If I could just get that label, then I could get her help.

When all the tests were finished, Hannah was diagnosed with anxiety, depression, obsessive compulsive tendencies, separation anxiety, attention issues, and sensory processing disorder. But there was no autism label (though sensory processing disorder is actually on the spectrum).

The diagnosis didn't give us anything new. It seemed they had simply read the information we gave them and regurgitated it back to us. I questioned the doctors about Hannah's social interactions, as she struggled greatly in this area. They said she did very well on the assessment of socialization; she knew exactly what to do in social situations. They commented that she did not keep eye contact but they thought it was because the assessor intimidated her. I told them she was very bright and knew what she should do, but didn't do it! They insisted she did not have autism. I was devastated – this just validated what the school had been saying.

I now know that there is power in the spoken word. In hindsight, I believe God protected Hannah by not allowing that label to be placed on her. Even though she had most of the symptoms of Asperger syndrome, a high functioning form of autism, God protected her from that label, too.

Personally, I felt I had hit bottom, but this wasn't the first time I'd felt that way only to find that the hole was deeper still and I would drop down again. It felt like a bottomless pit.

Right before this appointment, we had a night where my husband and I decided that the next time Hannah got upset, we would just "let her go" and see how long it would last if we simply ignored her. So the next time she began having a fit, we put the other kids to bed and sat on the couch, chatting. Hannah would run out, yell, scream and then run into our bedroom. She was not getting our attention and it was really making her mad. Finally we had a confrontation. She melted into a puddle and began crying hysterically, saying, "I'm sorry, I'm sorry!" All I could think was, "It's hard to control her at six; what will she be like when she is thirteen?"

THE TOLL ON A MARRIAGE

After that, the days became even longer. My husband was home less and less. He insisted it was because of work demands. While I knew this was partially true, I also knew it was because things were so bad at home. Don't get me wrong – he was always very supportive and helpful. The problem was that I would not let anyone else deal with Hannah. I didn't think anyone else could handle her, so I made him feel everything he did was wrong! So many times he would try to help and I would yell at him about how wrong he was doing things. Then I would step in and take over, because I had the mind-set that only I could do it! It was nasty, unhealthy and totally out of my control.

Things were deteriorating with Hannah's behavior, and our marriage was following close behind. Our relationship was getting more and more distant. I didn't feel like I even knew him anymore. Everything he did frustrated me and I felt totally isolated. We both felt like we had become roommates in the middle of a war zone. Every day seemed worse than the last and we had nowhere to turn.

NOT BY MY POWER

One Thursday night, when my husband was working late, I prayed, crying out to God once again. I told God I couldn't do this anymore. I hated my life, my marriage was a mess, and I felt like a terrible mother because there was nothing I could do to help my daughter. I just wanted to get off the world until it was all fixed.

I lay there on my bed with my eyes closed and God spoke to my spirit. He showed me that He would heal her. It was not going to be by my strength and the "work" of my hands, but through HIM. I had done everything I could do, but the situation was bigger than me. God would have to do it – the supernatural power of God would have to invade if my daughter was going to be healed.

At that point, I gave my daughter over to God for the first of many times. I asked Him to show me, through wisdom and revelation, how to help her. I knew none of the medications or doctors were going to help. God had a plan to heal Hannah and He had chosen me, as her mother, to seek Him to work it out. This is where the path to miraculous healing began.

Chapter 3

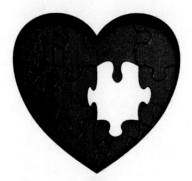

THE ONION:
REVELATION UNFOLDS

The counsel of the Lord stands forever,
The plans of HIS heart from generation to generation.
Psalm 33:11

The Lord knows our hearts, and my deepest desire was for Hannah to be healed, happy and free. The Lord surely was giving me the desire of my heart, even though in the midst of it, I couldn't see it. Up to this point, I was in a place of half-hearted daily prayer and crisis prayer. A crisis would hit, I would run to God, then go on in my own strength until the next crisis. As one author put it: I was jogging with Jesus versus running the race of a champion.

So I entered a new season. I began seeking God every day. I knew there was more to God than I was experiencing. I had seen glimpses, but I wanted to *know* this God I had been learning about since childhood. I started developing a real relationship with Him!

I had often felt hopeless, and many mornings were filled with fear about what the day would bring. But after crying out to God that

Thursday night, God became my new best friend. I began talking to Him about everything!

As a child I had desired to read the Bible, but it was like reading a foreign language – I hardly understood a word I was reading. Even in high school and college, I had tried reading it but always gave up because I didn't get it. I got up early Friday morning and opened my Bible to try again. This time I prayed and asked God to help me read and understand His Word. For the first time, I got it! A whole new level of understanding opened up for me. I comprehended every word of what I read and it applied to what I was going through.

That day I began the first of many journals that captured those precious times with God. I wrote this prayer:

Come Spirit of living water, fill me with more faith, more of You and Your Spirit. Strengthen my heart, Oh Lord, hear this prayer. You are the author and protector of my faith. You are the author of my life; reveal the plot to me so I may be obedient in my walk. Jesus, You are my only hope. You are faithful and true, the one and only GREAT LIGHT in this darkness. Come Jesus, be the head of me. Give me Your light for revelation, Lord of peace, bright and glorious morning star, my friend, my intercessor, come. Lord, thwart my plans and purposes. Show me the plans You have for me and for Hannah, because Your plan stands firm forever. I want to walk in Your firm plan, not my own. Your eyes are on me and my hope is fully in Your unfailing love. I wait for You. You are my helper and my shield. I trust in Your holy name! May Your unfailing love rest upon me as I put my hope in You.

Something inside me came alive. I felt hope for the first time in a long time. Little did I know that the answer to this prayer was right around the corner. The Lord was about to burst open the revelation that would bring healing to my daughter and peace to our family.

I shut my Bible as I heard my little Matthew waking up. It was time to start the day. What would it hold? We needed to be at church by 9am for MOPS (mothers of preschoolers) and it was always a challenge getting Hannah out of the house. However, the morning went pretty well.

The hope I was feeling dwindled as I drove and began thinking about everything again. How was *I* going to help my daughter if nothing was working? What hope was really there? By the time I got to church, I totally had talked myself out of any hope and was feeling defeated once again. How quickly and easily we allow lies to enter in over the truth of God!

A NEW DOOR OF HOPE

At the church, I was relieved to have a bit of a break and be with some other adults. I was pregnant with our fourth child and exhausted physically and emotionally. The kids were all checked into childcare and I was sitting with other women in a peace-filled room when Robin, the mentor mom, got up to pray for the morning.

After praying, Robin said she would be available at the back of the room if anyone needed personal prayer. I couldn't sprint back there fast enough. I told her what was going on with my daughter and what God had revealed to me. She prayed for my daughter, my family, and me – then she asked, "Have you ever tried the natural route?"

The moment she spoke it, I knew that it was a word from God. My spirit immediately lifted and something inside of me just knew that the words she was speaking were opening a new door of hope. I suddenly felt peace flood my heart. This was the wisdom and revelation I had prayed for just the night before – God was answering my prayer and beginning to reveal how He was going to heal Hannah.

"Huh?" I asked. "What is the natural route?"

Robin suggested a chiropractor to begin our journey into the natural world. A red flag flew up in my mind when she said *chiropractor*. I was raised in a home where we were not allowed near a chiropractor and were told they were all "quacks" and frauds. I didn't feel particularly confident with that advice, but this whole natural route sounded intriguing. She explained that the natural world consisted of the use of food, spinal alignment and supplementation to aid in healing the body. It all sounded good except for the chiropractor. But she made it sound like an integral part of treatment, so I decided to try it for myself first.

I was at the beginning of my fourth pregnancy and very ill. I had dealt with illness throughout all of my previous pregnancies, so I decided to try out the chiropractor and see if he could help me feel better. I thought that if he could help me, I would then bring Hannah.

When I saw the chiropractor Robin recommended, he told me that my gallbladder and liver were stressed due to my pregnancy and that with supplement support I should feel much better. Guess what? I took the nutritional supplements he recommended and I did feel better! I no longer needed to take the anti-nausea medication I had been taking. I didn't feel totally well, but I did feel much better.

The next week I took Hannah to see this Christian chiropractor. I was amazed at what he was able to tell me about my daughter in just one visit. He told me she had a yeast overgrowth in her stomach and food sensitivities to dairy and sugar. We were instructed to totally eliminate dairy, sugar and high fructose corn syrup from Hannah's diet. She also had major problems in her spinal alignment that compounded all her issues. Her liver was stressed so I was told to feed her lots of beets and lemons, as they strengthen the liver. Her immune system was compromised from the medications and nebulizer so, even though we did not eliminate these medicines at this time, she began taking flaxseed oil to boost her immune system. Who would have known that food could actually help in the healing process?

I left the office filled with hope. However, when I got home and looked in my cupboard, I was overwhelmed to realize that sugar, high fructose corn syrup (HFCS), and dairy were in EVERYTHING!

I called Robin, the mentor mom I was working with, because many years earlier she had gone the natural route and her daughter was healed of a life-threatening illness that the doctors said could not be healed. I thought, *If God did it for her daughter, He will do it for my daughter, too.* I was able to confirm this with Scripture – Revelation 19:10 says, "For the testimony of Jesus is the spirit of prophecy." The testimony was Robin's story of what Jesus did in her life and the Spirit of prophecy was telling me that what He did for her He would do for us because Jesus is not a respecter of persons (Romans 2:11). I was encouraged that this journey we were on would bring victory and freedom to us as well as others.

Robin said that our journey would be like an onion – we would slowly peel away one layer at a time. That's exactly what happened. We had already peeled off one layer – the medical world. The next layers were chiropractic, diet, supplementation, and spiritual – there were many layers to this big onion.

Robin became my lifeline, walking with me every step of the way. She told me of dairy-free alternatives and things for snacks that did not have sugar or HFCS (high fructose corn syrup) in them. I was so blessed by her! I went to the co-op to buy our new food. I must admit that I ended up abandoning my cart twice, leaving the store in tears, thinking, *That's $500 worth of groceries, more money than I've ever spent at once on food. I don't know how to cook it or if anyone will eat it!* So, again I talked with Robin, who gave me a specific list of foods. I went back to the store and bought only what was on that list.

We immediately saw that there was a huge connection between sugar/dairy and Hannah's behavior. Once Hannah began her new diet, I visited her teacher at school and explained what we were doing, and that Hannah could not have any food at school unless I sent it with her.

Hannah was doing great, until one day she got off the bus and the minute her foot hit the ground she began to cry hysterically. I walked out the door to meet her and asked if anything had happened on the bus. She said, "No." I asked if something had happened at school and again she responded, "No." I then asked what was wrong and all she could say was, "I don't know," and she buried her face in my tummy, sobbing. I gave her a big hug and we sat on the couch. I called her teacher to see if something had happened at school and she confirmed that Hannah had a great day. When my husband Paul got home from work it was almost 7pm. He walked in the door and she ran over to him and finally stopped crying. She had cried uncontrollably for almost three hours.

When Hannah finally calmed down enough to talk, I asked if she had eaten anything at school. She said that on the field trip the teacher had forgotten the snack I had specially prepared for her so she let Hannah have a graham cracker. I knew that was the culprit. Every time she had a hint of sugar or dairy her reaction was this intense.

911

On October 13th of 2006, Michael, our fourth child, was born. A week later Paul had a weeklong business trip so my in-laws, who are wonderful, came to help me out. We had just switched Hannah's medication from Lexapro to Zoloft and she was in her room having a total meltdown while all the other children were in their beds sleeping. My in-laws and I sat at the kitchen table listening to her. No one knew what to say. I then read the warning label on her medication. It said it could lead to depression, suicidal thoughts, and suicide. I read it out loud to my in-laws and said, "What in the world? I am giving her this stuff so she doesn't kill herself and this tells me that suicide can be a side effect. What is the point?" After reading that label, I was refueled – a new resolve hit me to really focus on how to get her off the medication, no matter what it would take.

We were now doing natural health, using medication, and seeing numerous doctors. Taking out the dairy and sugar did make the meltdowns less frequent and intense, but they still happened. They were now disrupting our lives for only an hour or so instead of two or more, and they were only happening a couple times per day versus four to five. And now Hannah was losing control in front of other people and in public places on a regular basis. She was no longer able to hold it all in until she got home.

It was hard to watch her go through this; she was tired and so were we. It seemed sugar and dairy were part of the problem but not the total solution. We needed the key to the next layer of this onion. I knew that answers would only come as God revealed them. I was counting on Him to give me the courage and strength to press on in the journey!

One night we were on our way to dance class and Hannah decided she didn't want to go. She became increasingly upset the closer we got to class. We pulled into the parking lot and she was determined not to go to dance. She was crying and screaming, "No, Mommy, no!" I parked and got everyone else out of the van. When I got to Hannah, she continued to sit there, yelling and screaming. I said, "Fine. I'm sick of this – we're going home."

Then she looked at me and said, "No Mommy, I want to go to dance." I told her that this was not the way to act and we were going home. I got everyone back in the van, slamming the door behind me. I started the van and saw Hannah had gotten out of her seat and was now lying on the floor, so I told her to get back in her seat and buckle up, which she didn't.

"Get in your seat now, or I will call the police," I told her firmly, explaining that it was against the law for me to drive with her on the floor and I could get into trouble. She got in her seat but as I started to drive away, she jumped from her seat again, grabbed the steering wheel and yelled, "I want to go to dance!" She was trying to turn the car around. I slammed on the brakes and said, "Sit down and buckle up now or I will call the police. It's illegal for me to drive if you're not buckled in." She shouted back, "Fine, call them!"

I sat there for a moment. I had learned in my teaching years that when you threaten with a consequence you must follow through. I had a brief moment of hesitation and then picked up my cell phone and dialed 911.

I explained that my daughter would not stay buckled in her car seat and asked if they would send an officer over to talk with her. They agreed and within moments two police cars showed up. Talk about a humbling experience! There I sat in the parking lot of dance class with two police cars pulled up next to me.

I explained to the officer what happened and said, "I basically want you to scare her so she stays buckled in her car seat." The officer nicely replied, "I'll talk to her but I'm not going to scare her, I want her to know that we are here to help her!"

The police officer was great. He talked to her about the importance of wearing a seat belt and listening to your mother! She quickly buckled up and we were off. She was mad at me for calling the police but she learned that I mean what I say and I will follow through. She has never unbuckled again!

A DIVINE APPOINTMENT

I was talking to a friend about my frustration regarding the lack of progress despite all the effort we were putting into it, wondering if it was all worth it. Her response was, "You should really go see Dr. Matousek. She's an awesome chiropractor." I just took the comment in and went on my way.

The next week at church, I was talking to our nursery director about my concerns (she was one of my prayer warriors through all of this). She also told me, "You should really go see Dr. Matousek. We love her."

On top of everything else, Michael had not slept for the first three weeks of his life. I took him into our chiropractor and he, too, directed us to see Dr. Matousek, a chiropractor that specialized in pediatrics.

This was now the third time in three weeks that this doctor's name had come up. Sometimes God needs to tell me something more than once before I recognize He is speaking! I called and met with her on Monday morning.

When I walked through the doctor's door, I didn't know I was entering a divine appointment. Not only would God use her to minister healing to my daughter, she would ultimately become one of my best friends. I went in and talked with her about my newborn son. She tested him and found he was allergic to gluten, which he was getting through my breast milk. I quit eating gluten and four days later he was happy and sleeping well!

THE POWER OF THE TONGUE

After finding the answer for my son, I went into an extensive history with Dr. Matousek about my daughter and her issues. One of the first things she said was that we should never talk about Hannah's issues or struggles in front of Hannah. I was blown away. All the other doctors would not allow me to discuss the issues without her being present! Every time I would tell them what was happening with Hannah, she was sitting there listening. I felt sick to my stomach but I had no other option. This was another confirmation that God had led us to this new doctor. It also launched me into a journey of learning about the power of the tongue.

In the early days when God was teaching me something, it showed up everywhere in my life. Dr. Matousek opened up the topic by sharing with me that there is creative power in our words. Every time we told the story in front of Hannah, she was hearing how wrong things were. We were instructed to declare (or speak) over Hannah only words of healing and life. Soon after this, our pastor gave a sermon on the power of the tongue. Then I heard a daily devotional on the radio and guess what it was on: "The Power of the Tongue."

I began noticing the things I was saying to Hannah and others. It was terrible! I quit saying negative things about Hannah's situation to her or anyone else other than Dr. Matousek. This was the first step I took in speaking life into our situation.

In Hannah's initial exam, she had a back scan and kinesiology (muscle testing). I learned that Hannah had severe issues in her upper neck, all of which affect neurological functioning associated with anxiety, depression and ADHD.

I also found out through muscle testing that there were 23 foods that we had to avoid. The doctor confirmed the massive yeast overgrowth and started Hannah on treatment for that. We took many vitamin and mineral supplements and went even a step further in regard to our already very careful diet – drastically changing it to eating only fruit, vegetables and meat. (At this point we removed all grains from Hannah's diet. However, as she healed from the inside out, gluten free grains were added back into her diet, along with many other foods. This strict diet was temporary and helped her body to strengthen and get rid of toxins slowly.)

I learned that Dr. Matousek was not only a wonderful chiropractor but also a woman of unshakable faith. She silently prayed for Hannah from the time we walked in the door, through her appointments, and throughout the day as the Lord would lead. I later found out that even her receptionist was praying during our appointments. As we became friends she told me the many things the Lord had shown her about Hannah, physically and spiritually, and how that had directed her treatment. It was SO cool and right on!

The beginning was tough. We (all four kids and myself) went to our doctor's office three times a week, minimum. On the doctor's days off, we often would end up at her house because if Hannah had an emotional episode, she wanted to see her. After a meltdown, Hannah would be totally out of alignment (vertebrates in a straight line) and sometimes all of her supplements would need to be changed. The doctor would align her and adjust the supplements and Hannah would stabilize. This went on for several months.

A New Resolve

Moving to a diet completely free from processed foods and eating only fruit, veggies, and meat birthed a new wave of determination within me. I knew this energy and drive was coming from God because I was so filled with peace and excitement about this new layer of the journey that would help my daughter. No matter how hard or overwhelming the journey was, I knew Hannah was going to be healed. God was with Paul and me and would give us what we needed to do the job. I began praying daily not only for Hannah's healing but for the wisdom and strength to do all we needed to do.

I cleaned out our entire pantry, got out every cookbook I owned, and created a menu and shopping list. I then took the credit card and went to a grocery store and co-op to buy everything we needed for Hannah's even stricter new diet – free from dairy, sugar, HFCS, MSG, additives, preservatives, corn, soy, maple syrup, and food colorings to name just a few. Cooking became my life, because everything we ate needed to be homemade. When we first started with dietary restrictions I began to make much of what we ate, but now it was even more drastic – there was nothing pre-made that was free from all the things we had to be free from! My kids became great kitchen helpers and grocery shoppers.

While my little ones took to the new diet with ease, it took months to develop ways to get Hannah to eat many of the new foods.

But, little by little, she ate more and more and became stronger and healthier. We prayed every day that God would give us a desire to eat the foods our bodies needed, and it helped! God gave me very creative ideas to get the kids to eat these new foods that they didn't think were too exciting. Instead of stress and battles over food, we made meal times fun. We gave foods silly names (e.g., macadamia nuts were called "baseballs" and cashews were "moonrocks") and played games to see if our tongue had changed its mind about new foods. We played with our food by making pictures and sculptures with it, then eating the "art" off our fingers. We did anything to get them to eat.

After a few months, I had a menu system for meals and snacks and I had a shopping and food preparation plan. Each week became easier and, as she continued to eat better, Hannah got stronger and began to heal from the inside out.

Our journey has been fueled by prayer and seeking God for His help and strength. When we cried out for Him to heal Hannah and show us what to do, He was faithful to answer. He led us to the right doctors (medical and natural), supplements, and diets – all critical pieces of Hannah's healing. From each doctor, we learned a piece of the puzzle and uncovered a layer of wisdom that would bring complete healing to Hannah. We then added supplementation, chiropractic adjustments, and modified diets, which revealed an even deeper level of healing.

The journey had brought some peace to our home and a hope was birthed deep inside of me that Hannah would be completely whole. We knew there was more work to be done, but we were now able to see a light of victory at the end of the tunnel. We were no longer just stabilizing or going backwards, we were making forward progress! Healing was coming, sometimes too slowly for us, but it was coming.

Chapter 4

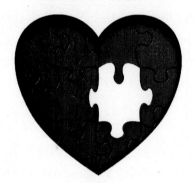

THE BATTLE IS WON

*But thanks be to God, who always leads us in triumph
in Christ, and manifests through us the sweet aroma
of the knowledge of Him in every place.*

2 Corinthians 2:14

In March of 2007 Hannah was eight, Lilli was five, Matthew was three, and Michael was six months old. Hannah was doing great. She was no longer experiencing meltdowns and other behavioral problems, as long as we had consistent spinal adjustments three times per week, made sure all her supplements were taken, and kept a very strict diet.

As a family, we were beginning to heal, so we decided it was time to take our first big family vacation. Our good friends, Matt and Sonya Bomhoff, had moved their family to Fort Worth, Texas, where they now served at Convergence, a cutting-edge Bible School and congregation with several hundred in attendance. We thought it would be a great time to just be together and reconnect. Little did I know that this trip would transform not only me, personally, but also our entire family forever.

After a long twenty-hour road trip, much of it in the midst of a powerful rainstorm that slowed us down for several hours, we finally arrived at our friends' house and reunited. It was so good to see them! While the kids ran off to play, we adults sat together and got caught up on all that had been going on with our families.

On Sunday we went to Convergence Church with our friends. It was an amazing experience. During the worship, I felt as if someone was putting a blanket around me. I didn't know what it was but it was so peaceful it made me excited inside. When the preacher got up to speak, he said, "Wow, the presence of God is so thick in here. Did anyone feel the weighty presence of God? It was like a big heavy blanket!"

I jabbed Paul in the ribs and said, "I felt that, exactly what he said." He looked at me with a weird kind of look but I was gripped – I wanted to know more about what was going on. I listened intently as this man talked about his ministry and told stories of miracles. He talked about how God was alive and active today and still heals just like He did in the Bible.

When the service was over, I was so energized that I felt like a new person. I knew God was with me and that He had been guiding our journey to Hannah's healing but I had never *physically felt* the presence of God before.

THE POWER OF DECREE

The next day my girlfriend Sonja and I went out for the day. As we were driving I said, "I'm fasting from coffee until Hannah is completely healed." I went on to tell her that Hannah was doing much better but still had a little way to go. She said, "When are you going to quit talking about her being healed and just take hold of the fact that she *is* healed and stand on it?" When I asked her what she meant, she explained that there is power in our words, thoughts and heart. She said if I believed with my heart and spoke it with my mouth, it would have power to solidify Hannah's healing.

We sat down and made a list of who Hannah was created to be – not behaviors *we* were seeing, but how *God* sees her. We also wrote down all the opposites for things we wanted to see go. For example, at this time Hannah struggled with reading; so on the list it said, "Hannah is good at reading, it is easy for her." The list ended up being two pages long. Sonja told me to decree, or read aloud, this list every day and have Hannah read it as well. I agreed, and a peace washed over me as I was filled with faith that Hannah was indeed healed. I said, "I believe Hannah is healed!" Sonja said, "Let's go have a coffee." We drove to the coffee shop and I have to say that it was the best coffee I had ever had!

The last stop for the day was Target. I quickly ran in to grab some diapers, when I had a revelation about life. As I was dashing through the store, I saw my past flash by – I saw my old house, I saw myself teaching in front of a group of kids, I saw my checkbook and my car. As I got to the check out, I heard in my mind, "What happened to you, where are you?" I began to laugh. I'm sure the lady at the register thought I was crazy.

I was still laughing when I got to the car. "What's so funny?" Sonja asked. "Well, I'm just wondering how I went from an independent woman with a career, my own house, my own checkbook, car and hobbies to who I am now. I don't know who I am. I have become so lost in this whole thing that I don't even know the balance of my checkbook. I think I need to rediscover myself." She began to laugh with me.

The years had flown by and I had totally lost myself in everything going on. With this revelation, I then made my own list of decrees about who *I* was and who God says *I* am. The first one was: "I am a competent person and I will see this through. God will completely heal Hannah and we will have victory." I began to declare it over myself every day, and my faith grew and grew.

On our way home I told my husband that once we got home, we needed to find a church like Matt and Sonja's where they believed in the gifts of the Holy Spirit and we could feel the presence of God, or we were going to move to Texas. He thought I was a bit crazy at that point!

We had been attending a wonderful church through the years and I was very grateful to those who had encouraged me and been part of Hannah's healing in the past few years, including MOPS (Moms of Preschoolers), my mentor Robin, and Cheryl and Deb, who first spoke to me of Dr. Matousek. I also had powerful prayer warriors who supported me during that time.

I now felt a pull, deep inside me, to learn more about what I experienced at Convergence Church in Texas. Something there was different! I wanted to totally embrace the supernatural of God – not only for us to receive complete healing – I desired intimacy with God. I had a new understanding of how Jesus was alive and active in me and I wanted more! I began to pray and ask God to show me more of Himself, and in the months that followed that's exactly what He did.

RELEASING HANNAH

Cast your burden upon the Lord and He will sustain you.

Psalm 55:22

About a year after our trip to Texas, I opened my journal and read an entry of something my daughter Lilli had prayed during that time: "Dear Lord, don't let the devil hurt Mommy's heart." I remembered that I was tucking in my little Lilli, who was five at the time she spoke those words – they cut right to my heart. I left her room and I felt a rush of all we had been going through and how consuming it had been, how much fear I had previously, and how I had grown so much to trust the Lord. My heart had been so broken through the events of recent years, and my little Lilli knew it.

Her words revealed how deep that pain really was. I had been stuck in the "tornado" for so long that I had not even stopped to feel what was going on in my own heart. First, for many years I had tried to heal Hannah on my own; then I began to seek God to help, but I had never given her (or any of my children, for that matter) fully to God. I tried but wasn't successful. My heart had been broken.

A few weeks later I was at a meeting for moms called, "Hearts at Home." The speaker talked about how our kids are a gift to us from God and that we must trust Him to take care of them. She said that we must let our kids go, and trust God. She then had us cup our hands and visually place our children in our hands. Then we lifted them up and dropped them in the hands of the Father. I did this with tears streaming down my face. I had a deeper revelation that my only hope was in the Lord alone, not in myself.

There had been so many visible improvements in Hannah! However, I was living in constant fear that it wouldn't last. I was afraid that it would all come back with even greater magnitude, and that the spiral of turmoil would begin again. Worrying about Hannah had become a way of life for me. I needed to surrender her to the Lord (as well as my other children).

Instead of worrying about Hannah, I needed to pray for her. I began to continuously keep my focus on the Lord and rejoice in what He had done, what He was still doing, and what He was going to do. I had to trust God to guard and protect Hannah, and all my children, and silence the wicked (1 Samuel 2:1-10).

After this act of surrender, I spent quite a bit of time giving Hannah to God and then taking her back again. It was a vicious cycle. One of my journal entries echoed this trend in my life as I tried to fully surrender my daughter to the Lord's care:

Forgive me, Father, for not running to you. Once again, I've let myself become overwhelmed instead of resting in Your love and peace. Forgive me for taking Hannah back into my own hands again and for not letting You work in her life.

As time went on, this happened less and less. The more time I spent with God and the more I got to know His heart, the more I trusted Him with Hannah and my other children. Through this relationship I was able to build trust and know that the best and only place for Hannah to be was in His loving hands.

After returning from Texas, we began attending a church that was fully functioning in the gifts of the Spirit. Since our previous church did not believe in the supernatural gifts of the Spirit, I found myself in an interesting place of wanting to make sure this new church was in line with the Bible, but I didn't know how to be sure, other than if it "felt" right. One day a friend of mine, who is the director of a very sound women's ministry, told me she was doing a teaching series for women on healing, prophecy and the Holy Spirit. I quickly signed up and found the Lord had created a bridge for me from where we had been to where we were going. I learned all about the gifts of the Spirit and what the Bible says about them. I was pleased to find out that our new church home, The House Church, was right on track!

At the healing class, a woman praying for me said into my ear, "You don't need to worry about Hannah – God's got her!" I was shocked! This lady did not know my daughter, our situation, or me. It was the first time I knew I had heard directly from the Lord through someone else. I later learned that one way God speaks to us is through other people. An amazing peace fell over me after that woman prayed, and for the first time I was able to *fully* surrender my precious daughter into the capable hands of the Lord.

RESTORED RELATIONSHIP

One of my fervent prayers was that there would be restoration between my daughters. Lilli has such a compassionate heart that whenever Hannah would lose control or get upset, she would try to help her sister. In the midst of a meltdown, her efforts to comfort would result in her getting hit, kicked, yelled at, bitten, etc., and they would *both* end up in tears.

Most of Lilli's first six years of life were filled with her sister having multiple meltdowns. I prayed that they would have a strong bond and great relationship as they grew up, but things had been so violent and verbally harsh between Hannah and Lilli that I knew that God would have to do a work in both of their hearts for this to ever happen. In 2006 I wrote in my journal, "Lord, I lift up Lil and Han. May they be bonded together in love; bring harmony to their relationship."

In 2008 the Lord instructed me to homeschool my girls and that one of the reasons was to bring healing to their relationship. That first year, you never would have known that God was at work. It actually seemed worse than ever! It took time and lots of prayer, but by the winter of 2009 we began to see the fruit of all those prayers. My girls now spend hours playing together and truly enjoy each other's company!

TEACH WHAT YOU'VE LEARNED

One spring day, I was sitting outside watching my children as they played together. They were enjoying each other, and giggles and laughter filled the air. I sat there watching them and thanking God for all the revelation He had given me about our daughter. I thanked Him for how peace was filling our home most of the time. I thanked Him for healing my daughter and family and giving me the strength for what He called me to do to bring forth healing.

I then asked the Lord, "What should I do now? My kids are happy, Hannah is healed, and the hearts of our family are in harmony." In His soft, quiet voice He said, "Go teach moms!" It swirled in my mind. I had taught kindergarten and first grade ... but moms? They were out of my league!

The next day, I called the Community Education office and explained the idea God had given me for teaching a class. They said, "Sounds great. Can you get a proposal to us by Monday?"

"Sure," I said, totally stunned. That was the beginning of *Kingdom Kids Nutrition*. Since that day I have been writing, teaching and cooking with moms (and even a few dads)!

As I began outlining my class, I asked God what He wanted me to teach. First, He led me to research the impact of food on our bodies. My eyes were opened to the lies and deception of many in the food industry. Secondly, I was to teach moms how to align their family's diet with God's plan so we can create strong warriors for His kingdom through smart choices and menu planning. And finally, I was led to create a support system of like-minded parents for fellowship and encouragement, providing the strength to press through as we implement God's design for healthy eating.

A FUTURE WITH PURPOSE

The Spirit of the Sovereign Lord is on me, because the Lord has anointed me to proclaim good news to the poor. He has sent me to bind up the brokenhearted, to proclaim freedom for the captives and release from darkness for the prisoners, to proclaim the year of the Lord's FAVOR and the day of vengeance of our God, to COMFORT all who mourn, and provide for those who grieve in Zion—to BESTOW on them a CROWN OF BEAUTY instead of ashes, the OIL OF JOY instead of mourning, and a GARMENT OF PRAISE instead of a spirit of despair. They will be called oaks of righteousness, a planting of the Lord, for the display of HIS SPLENDOR!

Isaiah 61:1-3 (NIV, emphasis added)

This Scripture is the backbone of *Kingdom Kids Nutrition* – it speaks to me on both a personal and professional level. Through the miraculous process with my daughter, I was healed of a broken heart and can now walk with others whose hearts are broken. I am filled with freedom, knowing that she can now live a life marked with joy and hope, not despair! Our family has been released from being held captive by the darkness of sickness. The Lord's favor was upon our lives and He brought comfort during the times I mourned for my daughter, praying for her to have a "normal" life.

As God healed Hannah, He bestowed on our family a crown of beauty instead of the ashes we had lived under. He has brought us the oil of gladness in place of the mourning we had felt for so long. God has poured out a spirit of praise and thankfulness in place of the despair that plagued us for years!

I now feel that we are oaks of righteousness, a planting of the Lord, for the display of His splendor – we have become a testimony of God's goodness.

God brought me through this process so that I may now walk alongside moms to help bring life and health to their families. I am called by God to proclaim freedom for people stuck in poor eating habits, giving them tools to easily move forward to natural health.

I want to stand with those who mourn for their struggling children and replace despair with the hope of our story. My desire is to see God work in the lives of each and every person, that they would be strengthened and walk in victory!

My people are destroyed for lack of knowledge.

Hosea 4:6

Our family was being destroyed until God revealed the knowledge which led to complete healing for my daughter and, ultimately, our entire family. The knowledge God has given me is the message of life and how to acquire it through good nutrition, supplementation, and alignment.

VICTORY - THE CALL

*And we know that in all things God works
for the good of those who love Him.*

Romans 8:28 (NIV)

God loves us so much! It was truly by God's right hand and the light of His face that we were brought into victory with Hannah. For that, I will praise His name forever. God, You are my King – it was You that decreed victory for Hannah. Through You we were able to push back the enemy and through Your name we trampled our foes! You, Lord, gave us victory! In God we make our boast all day long! We will praise Your name forever.

All those years I was praying for healing and that is exactly what I got. *Healing* is defined as "the restoration to wholeness." It took about nine years in total, but restoration has happened for my daughter. Many times I doubted my daughter was being healed but I continued to pray, expecting a miracle, something instantaneous. Part of me thought that one day my daughter would just wake up completely healed. God can, and does, do miracles in that way; but what He walked us through was a process of healing, restoration and wholeness.

Because of this process, I am now able to help others. Ours is a powerful story of God's love, goodness and faithfulness. Without the journey, there wouldn't be much of a story and I wouldn't have grown to know the Lord as I do now. God is not a respecter of persons – what He did for us, He will do for you, too. I call forth the supernatural healing power of God to each and every person that reads this story. I decree that you, too, will have victory!

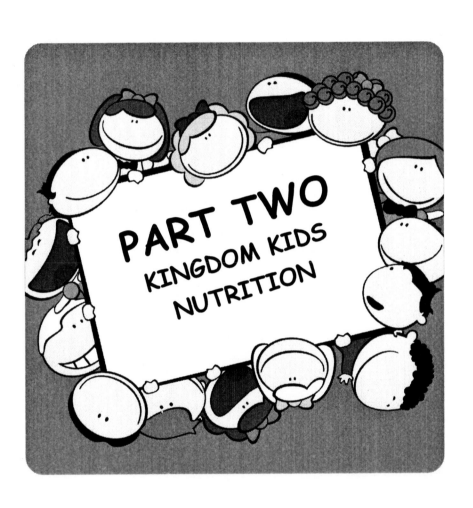

PART TWO
KINGDOM KIDS
NUTRITION

Chapter 5

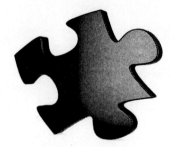

THE FOOD:

Back to Basics!

Through our journey, I learned what a powerful instrument food is! God made our bodies extremely strong and resilient; as we gave our daughter real, unprocessed, living food, her body began to repair and heal rapidly!

This section on food is a tool in the healing process. As you read the following information, please keep in mind that God is the one who supplies us with our health, not the food! We can use wisdom in our food choices, but ultimately God provides our health.

I want to share information I've learned to help you understand issues regarding our food supply and the effects of processing our food. My hope is that this information will help you to make better choices about what you select to eat and feed your family. So as you read, become informed but don't become legalistic about it. Use this as a guide to make smart dietary decisions. You're going to learn how God created food, and that eating food in its pure form is the best bet to give you and your family optimal nutrition and benefits!

Your body was created to function on the real, living food that God created. I define "real, living food" as any food that grows from the ground (like fruits and vegetables), eats from the earth (like cattle and chickens), or swims in the water (like fish). The American diet is far from "real," so hopefully this information will give you the desire and motivation to make the changes that will take back your diet.

Remember, it's a journey – a process that will not happen overnight. Choose one thing, tackle that and then move on to the next. If you try to make all the changes at once, you'll be overwhelmed and be tempted to quit!

It can be helpful to connect with other parents that have a similar interest in health and nutrition. You can form a group in your area and get together to share with each other what you're working on. You can hold each other accountable, share recipes, successes, and tricks of the trade.

There are twelve foods that I found really affected my daughter either positively or negatively. I began to research different ingredients and found that not only did they cause a problem for my daughter but have potential to cause health problems overall.

As I discuss these foods, you'll see which ones should be eliminated, which ones should be increased, and how your choices can impact your child's health as well as your own. There are many great alternatives that will keep your diet tasty as well as healthy! Be encouraged and know that I am praying for anyone who is reading this, that you will be given divine strength to take back your child's health through real, living food.

High Fructose Corn Syrup/Sugar

First, let's look at high fructose corn syrup (HFCS) and refined sugar ("table" sugar). In the article, "Sweet, but Sinister," Debra Ginsberg wrote that HFCS is the cheapest sweetener on the market –

much sweeter than sugar – so it takes a smaller amount for the same amount of sweetness. Amy Palanjian states in her article, "The Facts About HFCS," that the soda pop industry was one of the first to start using HFCS. Do you remember when the "super size" came into being? It was because of the use of HFCS. The restaurants were now able to sell a large soda that had HFCS in it for the same price as they used to sell the small soda that contained sugar. The 12 oz. soda made with regular sugar cost the same as a 24 oz. soda made with HFCS.

Did you know that the average person consumes 63 pounds of refined sugar, or its equivalent, per year? Grinsberg also states in her article that the consumption of HFCS increased 1000% from 1970 to 1990 and has further increased in usage 250% over the last fifteen years. The World Health Organization states that no one should consume more than 10% of their diet in sugar, no matter the source (natural: fructose, honey, molasses or processed: refined sugar, HFCS). That calculates out to no more than 200 calories per day from sugar for a 2,000-calorie diet. That's not much!

CORN

Another concern with HFCS is the current problem with corn in general. Corn is highly contaminated. When you see a sign or store label stating, "No GMO's," it means that the product has no genetically modified organisms – in other words: the product is in its natural form. Conventionally grown corn is very contaminated with GMO's. My naturalist doctor said that currently, conventional corn contains pesticides inside the DNA of the corn. Yes, that's right! The corn has been genetically modified so the pesticide is actually inside the corn kernel that is planted. Therefore, the bugs fly around, land on the corn plant, take a nibble and fall to the ground – the pesticide inside the plant attacks the nervous system of the bug and they fall dead!

This is great for the plant, but when we eat this corn we also ingest the pesticide. This has worked so well that there is discussion to put weed killer into the plant as well. So, future generations of corn will not only contain pesticide but they will genetically contain herbicide as well. Since all corn syrup comes from conventional corn, HFCS is highly contaminated.

The health risks that accompany HFCS (and sugar as well) are numerous. HFCS has been linked to the rising rate of diabetes. Our chiropractor told me that HFCS is not processed in the stomach, but rather in the liver, thus taxing the liver because it has to work harder to break it down. She went on to tell me that HFCS increases the release of triglycerides (fat cells), which lead to higher levels of triglycerides in the blood leading to a higher risk of heart disease.

HFCS also inhibits the release of Leptin, a hormone that regulates appetite. So, when you eat a product with HFCS, your brain doesn't register that you're full, due to Leptin not being released. As a result, you continue to eat and eat. Our kids are eating *many* products that have HFCS in them and they are eating too much because they think they are still hungry. This develops terrible eating habits, resulting in overweight/obese children who are malnourished!

In *The Kid-Friendly ADHD and Autism Cookbook*, Compart and Laake show the link between concentration problems, focus issues (ADD and ADHD symptoms) and highly emotional mood swings.

We saw this with my daughter. When we first started modifying her diet, she was accidentally given HFCS one time at school (slips usually happened at school). She came home and started to bawl. When I asked her what was wrong, it took her a very long time before she was be able to get a grip on herself to answer. When she finally calmed down enough to talk, we realized the culprit was a graham cracker!

HFCS is also hidden in foods as a preservative to extend shelf life and as a freezer burn preventative (Debra Ginsberg). Therefore, it is found in many NON-SWEET items. So, check those crackers and frozen foods before you buy them – they may contain corn syrup!

Some healthy alternatives for HFCS and sugar are: Turbinado (raw sugar), honey, molasses, xylitol, brown rice syrup, evaporated cane juice, sucanat (whole cane sugar), maple syrup, and maple sugar.

WARNING: *Do not* use artificial sweeteners in place of HFCS or sugar. They are very toxic, as we will discuss next!

ARTIFICIAL SWEETENERS

Artificial sweeteners are very dangerous! Sugar, even HFCS, is better than an artificial replacement. Artificial sweeteners are products such as NutraSweet, Aspartame, Splenda, etc. The problem with artificial sweeteners is that they are neurotoxins. A neurotoxin is a chemical that is toxic to our neurological system, specifically the brain.

Dr. Russell L. Blaylock, a professor of neurosurgery, published *Excitotoxins: The Taste That Kills* (Health Press, 1994) detailing specific damage done by the chemical aspartic acid found in aspartame. One of his main points was that excess aspartic acid is able to cross the blood-brain barrier and actually open your brain up to disruption.

Some of the reactions to aspartic acid coming from aspartame that have been reported to the FDA are: issues with focus, attention, emotions, depression and anything related to the neurological system.

It also opens up your brain to disease. Any disease that is floating around in your body is now able to infect your brain because the artificial sweetener has opened the blood-brain barrier. Many detrimental effects of artificial sweeteners have been reported to the FDA such as headaches and migraines, nausea, abdominal pain, fatigue, sleeping problems, vision problems, anxiety attacks, depression, and asthma/ chest tightness. Aspartame alone accounts for over 75% of the adverse reactions to food additives reported to the FDA (*Choose Life*, Seana Bukowski).

Our natural practitioner once told me that aspartame breaks down in the body as formaldehyde – obviously not good for the body!

Diketopiperazine (DKP) is a byproduct of metabolized aspartame. It alone has been implicated in brain tumors, uterine polyps and changes in blood cholesterol, as FDA toxicologist Dr. Jacqueline Verrett testified before the U.S. Senate.

There have been some studies that also link diet soda to the Gulf War syndrome. When I heard this from one of our doctors, I went home and did some research. I learned that the soldiers on active duty were given large amounts of donated diet sodas. The sodas were in plastic bottles and left outside in the extreme desert heat for days and even weeks. The desert heat caused the artificial sweeteners in the sodas to turn into formaldehyde, which was then ingested by the soldiers in large amounts. Even though not everyone agrees, there are a number of scientists who firmly believe that this was what caused the Gulf War syndrome – the toxins the soldiers were unknowingly putting into their bodies that effected their neurological functioning.

Monosodium Glutamate

Monosodium glutamate (MSG) is used in many processed foods. Many restaurants use MSG (be particularly aware of MSG in Asian restaurants). Dr. George R. Schwaltz, in *Bad Taste, The MSG Syndrome*, states that MSG is both a flavor and aroma enhancer and, for that reason, food companies in general have no intention of giving up MSG as an additive in their products. It's important that when you eat at restaurants, you request your food have no MSG. Also, check your labels closely. It's a very tricky ingredient to detect on the label because there are now many ways to label MSG. The following is an extensive – but not exhaustive – list provided by Dr. Schwartz of how MSG may be labeled on packaging.

+ Glutamate textured protein
+ Monosodium glutamate hydrolyzed protein
+ Monopotassium glutamate
+ Any protein that is hydrolyzed

- Glutamic acid yeast extract
- Calcium caseinate yeast food
- Sodium caseinate yeast
- Gelatin yeast nutrient

It is often found in the following as well:

- Malt extract flavors/flavorings
- Malt flavoring natural flavors/flavorings
- Barley malt natural pork flavoring
- Stock natural chicken flavoring
- Bouillon natural beef/chicken flavoring
- Broth seasonings
- Seasonings
- Carrageenan soy sauce
- Maltodextrin sauce extract
- Whey protein soy protein
- Whey protein isolate soy protein isolate
- Whey protein concentrate soy protein concentrate
- Pectin and anything protein fortified
- Anything enzyme modified

MSG has many similarities to artificial sweeteners because it, too, is a neurotoxin that crosses the blood brain barrier. MSG is actually an amino acid – which sounds like it should be healthy, but don't be fooled – this amino acid is one to stay far away from! MSG acts as an excitatory neurotransmitter, causing the nerve cells to discharge electrical impulses, firing rapidly, thus damaging and killing neurons with glutamate receptors by over-stimulating them (*Excitotoxins: The Taste That Kills*, Russell L. Blaylock, M.D.).

Food Coloring

Food coloring causes many problems in children. The nice thing with food coloring is that when you remove foods with HFCS from your diet, you usually by default remove food coloring, too. They are co-conspirators.

One of the main areas of concern around food coloring is for children who struggle with attention, focus, ADHD type symptoms, anxiety, or any neurological stress. One study showed that when food coloring was removed from the diet of children who were ADHD symptomatic, they significantly improved by 1/3 to 1/2 in the assessments of a typical improvement seen with medications. Just that *one* dietary modification of moving children away from "dead" food by removing food coloring, and moving them toward "real" food, made a huge impact. This little step could help many children avoid the ADHD label as well as the prescribed medication.

The UK has banned many artificial additives due to a study in Isle of Wright that showed detrimental effects of food additives (including food coloring) versus a placebo group.

There are specific food colorings that have been cited as a cause of behavioral and medical problems. For example, yellow dye #5 has been seen as a precipitating agent in asthma, eczema, hives, migraines, irritability, restlessness, and sleep disturbances ("Effects on Behavior and Cognition: Diet and Artificial Colors, Flavors, and Preservatives," Lucille Beseler, MS, RD, CS, LD).

Chapter 6

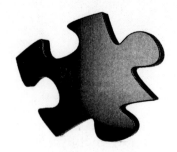

FATS:
THE GOOD, THE BAD, & THE UGLY

One of my favorite subjects to teach on is *good* fats! So many people have a false perception of fat being bad, when actually it is critical for optimal functioning in our bodies. It has a very important role in the human body and we're created to ingest a great deal of "good and beneficial" fats. We cannot survive and *thrive* on a low-fat diet. In this section we will look at which fats are "good" and should be consumed on a daily basis and which fats are "bad" and why you should stay away from them.

Fat does a body good! The following information is a summary from an excellent chapter on fats in the book *Nourishing Traditions* by Sally Fallon with Mary G. Enig, Ph.D. I would recommend that you read the chapter in full, because it's amazing! But, here is a sneak peek of how fats work with the body!

+ Fat provides our bodies with energy.

+ Fat is needed to convert carotene to vitamin A.

- Fats are the building blocks for our cell membranes, giving our cells stiffness and integrity to function properly.

- Fat slows down nutrient absorption so we don't feel hungry right after a meal.

- Fat is needed for mineral absorption to take place in the body.

- For babies and children it is *absolutely essential* for brain development and growth. Low-fat diets have been linked to failure to thrive children (Smith, MM, and F. Liftshuz, Pediatrics, Mar 1994, 93:3: 438-443).

Our culture tells us that all fats are bad but, as you can see, that's not true. So, the question is, where do we get these "good" fats?

- Good fats are saturated fats from quality meats and tropical oils such as coconut oil.

- Saturated fats are not trans fats and they are not hydrogenated.

- Saturated fats are stable, which means they don't go rancid when heated for cooking. (Rancid means that the oil releases free radicals, which cause cancer.)

- They are solid or semi-solid at room temperature.

- The best source of saturated fat is butter made from grass-fed cattle. The key is that the cattle have not been fed *any* grain. If they have eaten even a handful of grain, the beneficial qualities are no longer there.

Grass-fed butter is high in soluble vitamins A, D, K, and E, which are catalysts for utilization of the minerals we ingest in our food. Vitamin A and D specifically are essential for growth, healthy bones, brain development and a healthy nervous system. The Omega 3s and Omega 6 are in perfect balance, which is very important (we will discuss this in more detail when we talk about meat). Grass-fed butter also has a very powerful anti-cancer agent called CLA, which also builds muscle and prevents weight gain.

Grass-fed beef contain three to five times more CLA than grain-fed beef ("The Secret Sauce in Grass-fed Beef," Dr. Joseph Mercola). Grass-fed beef has good cholesterol in it, which is essential for growth and the production of steroids that naturally prevent cancer, heart disease and mental illness.

One of my daughter's main issues was a lack of good fat. At the beginning of our journey she needed large amounts of good oils to bring her neurological functioning back into alignment. For many months she took: barrage oil, flaxseed oil, olive oil, fish oil, and Lumina (another Omega-filled oil) on a daily basis. We also added coconut oil, grass-fed butter and beef to our daily diet and increased our intake of nut oils like peanut butter, almond butter, cashew butter, and sun butter.

Since our brains are basically composed of fat, it's essential to feed it good quality fats to ensure proper functioning. These quality fats come from grass-fed beef products, quality fish, and oils such as coconut, flaxseed and olive.

Once we began giving her oils, she gained the ability to control her emotions much better. Her meltdowns began to decrease, and her anxiety and OCD (obsessive/compulsive disorder) tendencies disappeared. She doesn't take as many oils now but still requires far more than the average eleven-year-old. That's just the way she is wired – her body requires a lot of oil to function at an optimal level. She eats lots of nuts, olive oil, coconut oil, grass-fed butter, fish and flaxseed oil on a daily basis and she weighs all of 65 pounds. So, needless to say, a diet high in good fats will not cause weight gain! Our entire family ingests a lot of good fats on a daily basis and none of us are overweight!

Other benefits to eating saturated fats include:

+ Lower lipoprotein [Lp(a)] levels, which determines proneness to heart disease.

+ A vital role in bone health because saturated fat is needed for calcium to be incorporated into the skeletal system.

+ Protects the liver from toxins.

+ Protects the digestive system from microorganisms that are harmful.

+ Enhances the immune system.

It is a total myth that saturated fats lead to heart disease. Actually, in a study it was found that 26% of arterial clogs were from saturated fat but the other 75% were from unsaturated fats – and half of those were from polyunsaturated fats, which is what the world is telling you to eat in place of saturated fats (Felton, CV et al, The Lancet, 1994, 344:1195).

MONOSATURATED FATS

You can tell if a fat is a monosaturated fat because they are liquid at room temperature, are relatively stable, and don't go rancid easily. They can be used when cooking with medium heat. You can find these fats in olive oil, almonds/almond oil, cashews, peanut/peanut oil and avocados. I use olive oil in all my cooking and baking, as it provides a great fat for my family in their everyday diet.

POLYUNSATURATED FATS

These fats are often called essential fatty acids or EFA's. They're called essential because your body can't make them – you must ingest them. There are two classifications to these polyunsaturated fats: healthy and unhealthy. The healthy oils come from flax seed and fish, while the unhealthy oils are from vegetables and should be avoided, especially when cooking.

All polyunsaturated fats are highly reactive, going rancid very easily and quickly. These oils are liquid at room temperature and should never be heated; keep them in the refrigerator where they will remain liquid.

Unhealthy polyunsaturated fats include: soy oil, corn oil, safflower oil and canola oil. Heating these oils cause free radicals to be released, which not only leads to cancer but also heart disease, immune system dysfunction, damage to the liver, reproductive issues, depressed learning ability, impaired growth and weight gain.

OMEGA OILS – ESSENTIAL BUT OVERLOOKED

Omega 3s and Omega 6 are essential fatty acids your body needs. The key with omegas is the balance. The American diet is high in Omega 6 and very low in Omega 3s due to the amount of processed food that floods our diet. This causes an improper balance between Omega 6 and Omega 3s in the average American person. According to Dr. Joseph Mercola the ratio should be no higher than 4:1.

The improper balance of Omega 6 to Omega 3s leads to making a person more prone to illness and disease. Everyone should take good quality fish oil. Nordic Naturals carries a great children's chewable – DHA Jr., which can be purchased online directly. Flaxseed oil in a smoothie or juice does wonders to boost the immune system.

These oils are also critical for optimal neurological functioning. If you or your child struggle with any neurological issues such as ADHD, anxiety, depression, OCD, autism, etc., omega oils are critical for the restoration and strengthening of the nervous system.

AVOID HYDROGENATED OIL

Sally Fallon gives a good word picture of how hydrogenated oil is created as she describes the making of margarine!

Cheap oil, such as soy, corn, cottonseed, or canola (already rancid from the heated extraction process) is mixed with nickel oxide (tiny metal particles), and then hydrogenated with gas at high temperatures. Soap-like emulsifiers and starch are then squeezed into the mixture to give it a buttery consistency – a gray substance results. This gray substance is then steam cleaned to remove the odor, bleached and dyed yellow. Strong flavors are added to make it have a buttery flavor.

You can't get much more processed than that! Stick with grass-fed butter; it's the healthiest choice.

Partially hydrogenated oils, also called trans fats, are actually worse than hydrogenated oil. It's dangerous because the digestive system doesn't recognize it as a toxin so it doesn't eliminate it from the body. Instead, it incorporates the trans fat into the cell membranes, causing your cells to become partially hydrogenated – changing the actual composition of the cell! It also blocks the utilization of essential fatty acids (EFA) in the body.

SUMMARIZING OILS

The way to keep your body in balance when it comes to oils is to have a diet high in good saturated fats such as nuts, coconut oil, and good quality meats. Use olive oil for all your cooking and baking needs – get rid of that canola! I know it's hard but you can do it. Also, make sure you and your family take a quality fish oil supplement to get those omegas in. Flaxseed is a must in every household because it has so many benefits!

Chapter 7

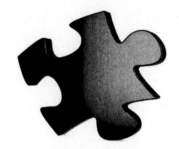

MEAT & DAIRY

Quality meat is essential for normal brain and neurological function. The brain needs Omega 6 and Omega 3 fatty acids which can be found in meats, especially in grass-fed beef (Dr. Joseph Mercola, Why Grass-fed Animal Products Are Better for You). Once again, the key word here is *grass-fed*. The ratio of Omega 6 to Omega 3s in grass-fed beef is 3:1. Dr. Mercola states that in conventional, and even organic grain-fed beef, the ratio of Omega 6 to Omega 3s is 20:1. This is also true of all dairy products that come from dairy cattle. When you ingest a food that has an Omega 6 to Omega 3s ratio that is higher than 4:1, you begin to have an increase in health-related issues, as stated earlier. Mercola continues by saying Omega 6 and Omega 3s play a significant role in the prevention and treatment of coronary heart disease, hypertension (high blood pressure), arthritis, cancer and inflammatory/autoimmune disorders.

We can put meat into three categories: grass-fed beef, organic meats and poultry, and antibiotic/hormone free meats.

GRASS-FED BEEF

Grass-fed beef is organic because the cattle are raised without grain, hormones or antibiotics – they were created to eat grass and only grass. Big farming and lack of land has led to feeding cattle grain, which entirely changes the composition of the meat. If we go back to the cow and its original God-given diet, it has *everything* we need in it.

Grass-fed beef is rich in fats that are proven to be health enhancing (good saturated fats along with balanced Omega 6/Omega 3s) and they are low in fats that have been linked to disease. These fats are in balance because when cattle eat how they were created to eat, they give us exactly what we need in the amounts that we need. So, when selecting the *best* meat to feed your family, choose grass-fed beef.

The only drawback is the high cost of grass-fed beef. In Minnesota, where my family and I live, you can only find this meat at your local co-op, and it's very expensive. However, I have found many farmers in the area who raise grass-fed cattle, and we buy our meat from them in bulk quantities (a quarter or half beef), making the expense equal to conventional beef in the grocery store!

ORGANIC MEAT AND POULTRY

Organic meat and poultry are free from hormones, chemicals, animal bi-products and antibiotics. These animals *do* consume grain but the grains are organic, which means they don't contain chemicals or pesticides. Animals that don't eat organically consume chemicals and pesticides through the grain and then pass them into the meat. So when selecting meat, this is a BETTER choice than conventional meat.

Antibiotic and Hormone Free Meat

Growth hormones are given to cattle to increase their size and their production of milk. This leads to increased hormones in dairy products as well as beef, which can then lead to early onset puberty (Dr. Sandra Steingraber, "The Falling Age of Puberty in U.S. Girls: What We Know and Need to Know").

Antibiotics are also a concern in our meat. Antibiotics are widely used to fight infection brought on from the cow producing far too much milk. This overproduction causes mastitis, which is then treated by antibiotics. Their living conditions, in which too many animals live in a small space, also contribute to the increase in illness and the use of antibiotics. The antibiotics are passed on in the meat and dairy, causing an overgrowth of yeast in our digestive system as we take in these products. This overgrowth (Candida) is on the rise and can cause numerous problems. Thus, your first step would be to buy meat that is hormone and antibiotic free. This is a good choice for your family.

Cold Cuts/Lunch Meats

Lunch meats are loaded with nitrates and sometimes sulfates – two ingredients that should be avoided at all times. Nitrates have been proven to cause cancer. The FDA allows them in meat because they say that nitrites cause cancer, not nitrates. However, according to our naturalist doctor, as the body breaks down nitrites, they are converted into the cancer causing nitrates, so the end result is the same. It's quite easy to find cold cuts that are nitrate free. A well-known brand that you can find anywhere is Applegate Farms.

The Question of Dairy

Whenever I tell people we don't do dairy in our family, their first response is, "What about your calcium?" Milk is actually not the best source of calcium for your body to absorb and use. In the article

"Choose Life, Eat Right," Seana Bukowski explains that cow's milk is high in phosphorous, and when phosphorous combines with calcium, it prevents calcium from being absorbed by the body. Also, the milk protein accelerates calcium excretion from the blood through the kidneys, causing your body to excrete calcium instead of utilizing it. The article goes on to say that it *is* possible to obtain all your calcium from dark green vegetables.

The best sources of calcium are dark green leafy vegetables such as romaine lettuce, kale, collard greens and similar, as well as other green vegetables, including broccoli or Brussels sprouts. God created these vegetables to have the synergy of vitamins and minerals needed to get maximum benefits for your bones. For example, a leafy lettuce, like romaine, has the perfect balance of calcium and vitamin D, allowing for ultimate absorption.

One doctor told me that a single leaf of romaine lettuce has more absorbable calcium in it than an 8 oz. glass of milk. Wow! That's when every member of our family began eating a leaf of romaine a day with peanut butter, rolled up like a wrap. That's how I introduced lettuce into our family. Now we have salads daily, and my five-year-old can out-eat me when it comes to salad.

CHEESE

Processed cheese contains emulsifiers, extenders, phosphates and hydrogenated oils, all things we should avoid. So, when we went dairy free, I went on a quest for edible and tasty cheese alternatives. Soy and rice didn't cut it for us, but I found goat cheese and we love it – we discovered a whole new world! Not only is there the traditional crumbled goat cheese, there is also tomato/basil and herbed goat cheese, mozzarella, cheddar and any other kind of cheese you need, just in goat variety.

Goat cheese is traditionally known as a dairy product. However, according to Dr. Alan Greene, the chemical composition in goat's milk is the most similar to human breast milk and therefore much easier to digest. (Dr. Greene is the Clinical Professor of Pediatrics at Stanford University School of Medicine, an attending pediatrician at Packard Children's Hospital, and a Senior Fellow at the University California San Francisco Center for the Health Professions. [drgreene.com])

The goat cheeses we use are also usually raw, so you get the nutritional benefits that are eliminated in cows' milk due to pasteurization. As we acquired the taste for it, we began to use it in all the ways we previously used dairy-based cheese. We also found that Pecorino Romano cheese – a sheep-based cheese that tastes like Parmesan – was also fine for our family.

MILK

We took dairy out of our diet due to my daughter's severe allergies. This was a huge issue for her but, as I researched dairy, we decided it best for the entire family to be dairy free.

Compart and Laake, (*The Kid-Friendly ADHD and Autism Cookbook*), state that the four most common food allergies are to milk, wheat, soy, and corn. Thus, I learned that dairy is one of the four highest allergens.

Another concern with milk is the diet of the cattle. Often they are fed soybean meal and grain with pesticides in them, contaminating the dairy with soy, pesticides and antibiotics, which are passed on to us when we drink the milk.

Hormones are widely used in the milk industry. The reasoning is simple – it boosts sales. A cow that is given hormones produces 10-25% more milk per day than the average cow. It's cost effective, but these hormones end up in the dairy products.

As we've discussed, these cattle often suffer from numerous infections and are given antibiotics. Just like they end up in the beef, they also end up in the milk, cheese, and yogurt ("Does Milk Really Look Good On You? Don't Drink It!" Ingri Cassel).

Cassel states in her article that cow's milk can cause diarrhea, cramps, bloating, gas, gastrointestinal bleeding, iron-deficiency anemia, skin rashes, asthma, acne, diabetes and ear infections. Our naturalist doctor told me that dairy is the *primary* cause of *ear infections* in children. This was supported in the articles I read on dairy and in my own experience. Since we quit dairy we have only had two ear infections, both after exposure to dairy. My oldest, who lived on antibiotics for the first three years of her life due to ear and respiratory infections, has been off them completely since we quit dairy!

PASTEURIZATION

Milk is very difficult to digest because the enzyme our bodies need to digest it is destroyed in the pasteurization process. Pasteurization really wreaks havoc on our dairy supply. In Cassel's article she says that a calf fed on pasteurized milk will die within 60 days.

Pasteurization:

+ Totally alters the milk chemically. It alters the amino acids lysine/tyrosine, making them less available for absorption.

+ The heat of pasteurization promotes rancidity of fatty acids, destroys the vitamins in the milk and reduces the concentration of minerals in the milk.

+ Causes strain on the pancreas because it needs to produce the missing enzymes killed in the pasteurization process.

+ Strips Vitamin D from the milk and synthetic vitamin D, which is toxic to the liver, is put back in.

+ Removes butterfat from our milk, which is critical to absorb any vitamins and minerals that might have survived.

("Don't Drink Your Milk" and "Choose Life, Eat Right," Seana Bukowski).

Raw dairy products are not pasteurized and are usually organic. They contain the enzymes we need to break down and utilize the benefits of dairy and also a bacterium that protects us against any pathogens that may be in the dairy. Raw milk is the *best* choice for milk but it's illegal to sell in the United States for human consumption. The only source of raw milk is a farm. However, raw cheese is available and it's the best choice if you're going to consume dairy from cattle. Your local co-ops will carry the raw cheeses.

Chapter 8

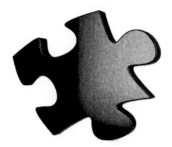

PURE FOOD

Living food brings life – Dead food does not!

Dr. Don Colbert

Health, wellness and life come from eating real living foods that grow from the ground, graze from the earth or swim in the water. Dead food usually comes from a bag or box, is highly processed, and brings illness and deteriorating health.

When deciding how our family was going to eat, I decided on the 80/20 rule. We eat 80% living food and 20% other foods. We also use the good, better, best rule. For example: It's *good* to eat Pea Crisp snacks (from a bag), it's *better* to eat frozen peas, and it's *best* to eat fresh peas. The closer you can get to the real food, the better. The more removed you are from the original food, the worse it is for you.

PURE WATER

The following is a summary from the chapter on water in the video series on water by Dr. Colbert, *The 7 Pillars of Health*:

The government has identified 2,000 chemicals in our drinking water: pesticides, drugs, hormones from birth control pills, antibiotics, pain killers, antidepressants, chlorine, fluoride, shampoo, etc.

I will highlight two that pose great risks: chlorine and fluoride. Chlorine destroys nutrients the body needs: vitamins A, B, E, and fatty acids. It has been linked to cancer, miscarriage, birth defects and spina bifida.

Fluoride has a similar structure to calcium. Therefore, if you have too much in your body, your body reads it as a calcium molecule and puts it into your bones. Thus, instead of strong bones built of calcium, bones are being weakened by the infiltration of fluoride.

What water to drink? The most inexpensive way to remove basic contaminates is a carbon-based filter like a Britta. If you're interested in bottled water, The International Bottled Water Association web site has a complete list of water sources. Dr. Colbert also has a bottled water list in his book, *7 Pillars of Health*.

Water is vital to good health and optimal brain functioning! The body is made up of 70% water. Muscles are 75% water, brain cells 85%, blood 82%, and bones 25%.

The brain uses water to manufacture neurotransmitters like serotonin, a well-known contributor to feelings of well-being. Water is needed to produce hormones that are made in the brain, including melatonin, which prevents ADD. Ample amounts of water improve the attention span. Make sure your kids drink water at school, especially before a big test or when they are studying. Hydrated brains function at a much higher level!

An article from the Kids Health website, "Why Drinking Water is the Way to Go," supports the many other benefits of water:

- It's the main component in lymph, which is what keeps your immune system strong and helps us fight off illness!

- Water – not cold – aids in digestion. (Cold water prevents the stomach acid from working effectively.)

- Water is needed for cells to properly function.

- Water improves memory and reduces the risk of Alzheimer's, Multiple Sclerosis, Parkinson's and Lou Gehrig's Disease (Dr. Colbert, *7 Pillars of Health*).

- As you go about your day, you lose two quarts of water. If you're thirsty, you're already one quart low.

- 80% of headaches are caused from dehydration.

- Caffeine and sugar steal water from your system. So if you consume caffeine and sugar, make sure to increase your water consumption.

- *Never* drink bottled water that has been sitting in a hot car or when you know the plastic has been warmed in any way, because heated plastic releases toxins.

Each day you and your children should drink half your body weight in ounces. So, if your child weighs 60 lbs, he/she should drink 30 oz of *pure* water per day. You can't add anything to it. Tea, coffee, lemonade or other flavored drinks don't count. Liquids that have water in them do not count for your water intake. Each day your water intake should be 100% water only! Our doctor says that even putting a slice of lemon in your water tells your body to process the water as a food substance, not a hydrating substance.

GLUTEN AND WHOLE GRAINS

As a whole, our country does not consume enough fiber. One way to increase the fiber intake is to eat more whole grains. Whole grains are less processed and are considered complex carbohydrates. They are absorbed by the body slowly and they stabilize blood sugar. They are very good for you, as opposed to simple carbohydrates, which are absorbed quickly and cause a quick spike in blood sugar.

Refined grains – like white flour – are stripped of nutrients and void of nutrition. They are a simple carbohydrate and should be replaced with hearty whole grains.

Gluten became a huge issue for our family, especially my youngest son. Gluten is any food item containing wheat, rye or barley. Gluten allergies and sensitivities are on the rise. One reason is that gluten is in *everything*, from vinegar that is in every condiment to the use of it as an anti-caking agent.

Another reason is that people love their soft bread, so scientists have been genetically modifying the wheat plant so that it contains more gluten, creating a wheat bread that is softer. However, this causes even more gluten exposure, creating food sensitivities in some people from overexposure. Because of this, it's good to mix up the flours you use in your home. The recipes in this book use a variety of flours so you will be able to easily do this for your family.

Chapter 9

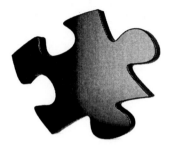

LABELS & SMART TIPS

I found most of the following information on labels from the University of Michigan Health Systems website – from an article called "Organic Food" and an article on meat labeling by Laura Everage called, "What's in a (Meat) Label – Is Your Free-Range Chicken Really Roaming Around?" Below is a summary from these articles to assist you in smart shopping!

When you shop for healthy foods the first thing that you need to know is how to read a label. Many labels are misleading marketing ploys to get you to buy something that looks healthy but actually is not!

Reading ingredient labels can get confusing and overwhelming. There are three questions I ask myself that drives my decision to select or reject an item:

1. Can you pronounce the words on the ingredient list or are there unfamiliar ingredients in the label? If you can't pronounce it, or if you can pronounce it phonetically but have no idea what it is, it's best to leave it on the shelf. You should be able to clearly read every ingredient and know what it is.

2. Does the label reflect the same ingredients you would use to make the food item from scratch? For example, if you're buying a loaf of bread the ingredient list should look something like this: whole wheat flour, yeast, water, and honey (or sugar).

3. Are there far too many ingredients in the list? When the list of ingredients takes up most of the packaging, then it is something to leave at the store.

Using these three questions can make looking at an ingredient label very simple. You want to purchase food products with ingredient labels that are short, reflect how you would make it in your very own kitchen (if you have the time and energy), and contain words you can pronounce and understand.

Another area where you need wisdom is in knowing what the packaging labels actually mean. Just because something looks and sounds healthy doesn't necessarily mean it is!

ORGANIC

What does "organic" mean on a packaging label? According to the United States Department of Agriculture (USDA):

+ If a product is labeled 100% organic, then by law there can't be any synthetic ingredients in the product – it actually is 100% organic.

+ If the label has the USDA seal on it, then 95-100% of the product must be organic.

+ A label that states "Made with Organic Ingredients" must have 70% organic ingredients and the other 30% must come from a list that has been approved by the USDA.

ALL NATURAL

Don't get tricked by the "Natural" or "All Natural" label. The USDA has not set a standard to regulate "natural" foods. This is just a marketing ploy, and the product could contain artificial colors, synthetic ingredients, preservatives, or chemicals. Read the ingredient labels carefully on all natural-labeled products to make sure they are truly a healthy choice. If it's a meat product, it's not supposed to have artificial flavors or colors, chemicals, preservatives, or synthetic ingredients – but the claims are not checked or regulated by the USDA.

LOCALLY GROWN

"Locally grown" foods are foods that have come from the area in which you live. These food can be organic or not (conventional)! The great thing about them is that they are grown in close proximity and contain many nutrients that are lost in foods that are shipped from a long distance.

CHEMICAL/PESTICIDE FREE

"Chemical-free" or "pesticide-free" foods are exactly that – free from chemicals and pesticides. This term is used a great deal at local farmers markets. Many times small farmers who do not have the resources to become certified as organic will opt to sell their product as chemical/pesticide free. They are basically organic but are not regulated or certified by the USDA. In this case I always make sure to know the farmer and farm to ensure that I am getting quality and truly chemical-free food. You can also check with your store's distributor – they will have all the information you need to ensure quality.

FREE RANGE

On many meat products, especially poultry, you will see labels that read, "free-range" or "free roaming." These products are usually *very* expensive. The USDA requirements for a free-range/free roaming animal are simply that the animal has an undetermined amount of daily outdoor access. So, the animal can be fed whatever the farmer wants to feed them, and when they go out, it may be a little pen with no real food for them.

A true free-range animal should be able to roam freely and eat only what they are created to eat. For cattle that would be grass and for chickens that would be grass, bugs and dirt! Many free-range animals are fed conventional diets containing pesticides and antibiotics, among other things.

I will only spend my money on free-range if I know the farmer and have seen with my own eyes that the animals are really roaming around eating what they were created to eat.

HORMONE/ANTIBIOTIC FREE

Another meat label that you want to watch for is "Hormone and Antibiotic Free," meaning that the animal has been raised on a hormone- and antibiotic-free diet. This labeling is used most with cattle and chickens. With beef you want to make sure that you buy your meat free from hormones and antibiotics. Any beef labeled in that way will ensure that you get quality meat free from those things.

However, chicken is a different story. It's illegal to give chickens hormones – therefore *all* chicken is hormone free. There was a chicken company that was injecting their eggs/embryos with antibiotics and then saying that the chickens were "raised" without antibiotics. Well, the chickens still had the antibiotics in them so the company had to remove the "raised without antibiotics" labeling from their products. When looking at labels on chicken, make sure it reads antibiotic and hormone free (not *raised antibiotic free*).

GRASS-FED

Grass-fed is a label usually found on beef. It is the USDA label that means a cow has been fed a grass-only diet. However, there is a practice in which a farmer will feed cattle grass until the last two weeks before butchering. In the last two weeks, the farmer will fatten up and tenderize the beef by feeding the cattle a corn-based grain, which enhances the flavor at the expense of all the nutritional value of the meat. When cattle are finished on grain this way, beef loses the good omega fats and the CLA that prevents cancer.

GMO Free

"GMO Free" is on many products these days. GMO stands for Genetically Modified Organisms. What this means is that the DNA of the product has been altered in some way. An example of this is when a scientist modifies a vegetable by incorporating herbicides or pesticides into the DNA of the vegetable thus making it resistant to bugs and weeds. GMO also can affect the growth and nutritional value of the vegetable. It's a good idea to stay far away from GMO products. The most common are corn, soy and wheat.

Choosing Organic or Conventional

What is the difference between organic and conventional farming practices? When I initially walked into a food co-op, I was intrigued and overwhelmed. The first big topic I had to address was the difference between organic and conventional. I quickly learned that conventional just meant the farming practices of large-scale farming. We will begin there.

Conventional Farming

Conventional farming is where any produce not labeled "organic" comes from. The farming practices of these large-scale commercial farms are very different from the organic farmer. Conventional farmers apply chemical fertilizers to the soil to expedite the growth and size of their crops. One major problem with this is that the plant grows so quickly it is unable to absorb the nutrients needed to make the plant a quality food source. Thus, produce grown in this way is often deficient in vital nutrients.

The conventional farmer also uses synthetic herbicides to control the growth of weeds in their fields. Many of these commercial farmers have their own personal gardens for their families, because they know the detriment to their health by consuming the produce contaminated by chemicals.

Jeffery Moyer, chair of the National Organic Standards Board, was quoted in *Prevention* magazine with this powerful testimony:

> *"Root vegetables absorb herbicides, pesticides, and fungicides that wind up in soil. In the case of potatoes – the nation's most popular vegetable – they're treated with fungicides during the growing season, and then sprayed with herbicides to kill off the fibrous vines before harvesting. After they're dug up, the potatoes are treated yet again to prevent them from sprouting. Try this experiment: Buy a conventional potato in a store and try to get it to sprout. It won't,"* says Moyer, who is also farm director of the Rodale Institute (also owned by Rodale Inc., the publisher of Prevention magazine). *"I've talked with potato growers who say point-blank they would never eat the potatoes they sell. They have separate plots where they grow potatoes for themselves without all the chemicals."*

The use of these harmful chemicals leaves the food tainted with a residue that can be harmful to humans. Dr. Mercola, in his article with Rachael Droege, "Why Do You Need Organic Food?" states:

> *The Environmental Protection Agency (EPA) considers 60% of herbicides, 90% of fungicides and 30% of insecticides to be carcinogenic (cause cancer) ... Pesticides can have many negative effects on health including: neurotoxicity, disruption of the endocrine system (hormones), carcinogenicity and immune system suppression. Conventional produce tends to have only 83% of the nutrients that organic contains.*

In the article "10 Reasons to Go Organic," Mercola and Droege state:

> *The scientific community is getting more concerned about the effects of small doses of pesticide exposure, especially in critical*

periods (fetal and childhood). They can have long lasting effects. It is advised that shoppers should minimize exposure to pesticides whenever possible. Washing and peeling may reduce but not eliminate exposure.

ORGANIC FARMING

A quick definition of organic farming is – the Creator's gardening. It is back to the basics of how farming should be done. Organic farmers feed and build the soil with natural fertilizers, such as cattle manure or compost, and rotate crops to maintain optimal soil nutrients. To control weeds, they use tillage, hand weeding, crop covering, and mulches – and they use natural predators and barriers to control insects, thus keeping the produce free from chemicals and pesticides. This type of farming is more time and labor intensive, so it adds some additional cost to the consumer.

SMART TIPS

I must state that it's better to eat conventional produce than none at all; it's better to eat conventional produce than rotten organic.

When I first learned about the healthier benefits of organic, I became totally rigid about it – if it wasn't organic I didn't buy it. I was unaware that there were ways to reduce chemical exposure when organic was not available.

One time I stopped at our local grocery store and there was just one very wilted organic romaine lettuce. I grabbed it, thinking I could salvage enough for dinner. As I walked to the cash register, I passed the beautiful conventional romaine lettuce. I glanced at my very wilted lettuce and proceeded to pay for it. When I got home I scraped together a limp but organic salad.

The next day I was talking to Robin, my mentor, and we were discussing the whole idea of organic versus conventional produce. She said, "Well, conventional is better than *rotten* organic." I just had to laugh, thinking back to our "icky" salad from the night before. I do try to provide as much organic produce for my family as possible. However, when in a squeeze, some is better than none.

THE DIRTY DOZEN

The Environmental Workers Group is a watchdog group that is always testing produce for contamination. On their website (food-news.org) they keep an updated list of the "Shopper's Guide to Pesticides" which lists the "Dirty Dozen" – the 12 foods contaminated with the highest amount of pesticides. It also lists the cleanest 15 foods that are lowest in pesticide concentration.

The first thing you can do to reduce your pesticide intake is to buy the Dirty Dozen organic. By doing so, you will significantly reduce your pesticide intake. If you only buy these twelve organic and the rest conventional, you will barely notice a difference in your grocery bill. Most grocery stores now have an organic section in which you can usually find these common twelve food items. I'm not going to list them, due to the fact that they change slightly from time to time. My suggestion is to go to the website, print out your own copy and carry it with you until you get to know them by heart.

WASHING

Another way to lower exposure to chemicals with conventional produce is to wash it thoroughly. There are different sprays you can use to wash your produce. Make sure to always remove any outer layers of leaves from conventional produce before you prepare it. Peel all the produce that you can, if it's conventional. However, if it's organic always serve it washed well, but retain the skin/peel on the produce because it carries most of the fiber and nutrients of many food items.

THE 80/20 RULE

If possible, in your diet allow 80% of what you consume to be living real quality food (organic); the other 20% can be of your choice (conventional). Our bodies are designed to be resilient and we really can do this without being legalistic about it.

Good, Better, Best

I use the Good, Better, Best idea when we travel. At home I can provide all the "best" options for my family. However, once we hit the road my choices become limited and I must decide from what I have in front of me. For example, at a restaurant instead of my children getting the kid's macaroni and cheese or chicken nuggets, we will order a steak or salmon dinner and split it between two of them. I then tend to spend about $15 for a meal instead of $5, but they split it and their meal was salmon, baked potato, and broccoli. A much better option than mac and cheese and fries! I am willing to pay the extra money.

Go and Slow

This is how I help my kids to make smart choices with snacking. I have two different bins. One I labeled GO – these are anytime snacks. The kids don't need permission to eat foods from the GO bins. I have one in the pantry and one in the refrigerator at their level, so they have free access. Grazing throughout the day is better than three big meals, so I encourage my kids to do this; it just must be truly healthy. The bin in the fridge has apples, carrots, celery, oranges, etc. The bin in the pantry has nuts, pretzels, raisins, mixed nuts and craisins, dried fruit, nut bars, etc.

We also have a SLOW bin in the pantry, which is not accessible to them – they can't reach it. This is our "treat" bin, and they must have permission to go into it. This would contain things like granola-type bars, organic corn chips, etc.

The kids quickly learn the difference between a snack and a treat and learn to make their own healthy food choices. As they get older, they realize they can eat anything in the GO bin, as much as they want, and they don't have an issue with weight or lack of energy, since they are eating real living foods that their bodies utilize!

Affordable Healthy Eating

Many shy away from eating organic or even healthy foods because of the cost factor. That's how I thought at first, but I learned that if I shopped wisely I could eat organic and healthy foods for about the same amount of money as conventional foods. Here are some tips that helped me really trim down my grocery bill.

Less Meat

The first thing is to eat less meat. This is overall a healthy practice. Even though meat is essential for our bodies, we can definitely cut down without any negative impact to our health. Start by having one vegetarian meal per week. You can make spaghetti with vegetables (pureed if need be) instead of meat, a veggie chili, bean and rice burritos, or a pasta dish. Once you and your family realize you can enjoy these meatless meals, you can increase to a couple of times per week.

Dirty Dozen

When you begin buying organic, start with the "Dirty Dozen." You will not notice a big difference in your grocery bill by purchasing these items organic.

Buy Produce in Season

When you shop the co-op instead of the traditional grocery store, you quickly learn the growing cycle of foods – what is in and out of season. For example, in the summer organic strawberries cost about $2.99 a pound – about the same as the conventional strawberries. However, in the winter when strawberries are out of season, organic strawberries run about $7.99 a pound while conventional strawberries will only go up to maybe $3.99 a pound. So, if you want out-of-season organic produce, your best value is to buy it frozen.

God has created our bodies to be in sync with the growing seasons. I have noticed that our bodies need different foods in different seasons to stay strong and healthy – it is all by God's design. In the summer you need berries, lots of raw vegetables, and grapes. And in the summer, the co-op is filled with these yummy foods at a very competitive price. In the winter, your body needs more root vegetables, less raw and more cooked vegetables, squash, apples, and oranges. And in the winter the co-op is filled with these types of vegetables at very competitive prices with conventional foods.

It's best to buy the produce that's in season to maximize your health but if you just can't live without strawberries in the winter, buy them frozen and you won't break the bank!

Farmers Market

Farmers markets are the prize jewels in regard to organic eating. When I go to the farmers market, I buy from a few farmers that I know are pesticide- and chemical-free. Always ask if they spray or use chemicals. I have found that most say no, which is not always true, but you can tell by looking at their produce. If it looks too good to be true, it is. I examine the tomatoes at a farmer's stand and if they have those little brown "bug bites," I know the farmer's produce is pretty clean. Keep walking if the tomatoes are big, bright red and without spots.

Local Farm Groups

Local farm groups are another option to get affordable organic produce. You pay the farm for the season, and each week you pick up your fresh produce at a local drop site. Be sure to research the farm carefully to make sure they have a good reputation in quality produce.

Buy in Bulk

Buying in bulk is another great way to make healthy eating affordable. Many areas have buying clubs where you buy in bulk with others, sharing the cost and the food. Your local co-op or the Internet will have information on a bulk-buying club in your area.

Another option is to become a member at your local co-op. They usually give a discount if you buy in bulk. The store where I shop gives a 10% discount on all cases you order, so the savings add up quickly. A great thing about the co-op is that when you join, you become a part owner, and at the end of the year you get a check based on what you spent. I usually get one weeks' worth of groceries back each year.

Your savings are maximized if you use a menu planning system to create a menu based on what is on sale for the month. Each month the co-op has a sale flyer for you to easily use in your menu planning.

RESOURCES

Trader Joe's is a great resource for getting some good deals on organic and healthy food choices. Whole Foods stores have their own brand of organic foods called "365 Organic". Their brand is usually a bit cheaper than the name brand products but do not compromise quality. Costco is also beginning to carry more organic, making this a good place to start as you transition into a healthier lifestyle.

Growing your own produce is also a great money saver. Does that sound overwhelming? Even an herb garden started in the window will save you money. We have a little plot in our backyard; the kids love to be part of the gardening process. Make it a fun family project. It's great family time and the kids will eat what they grow!

Another money saving tip is to have a realistic view of how much food kids actually will eat compared to how much food you serve them at each meal.

PORTION SIZES

When I learned that I was expecting my kids to eat far more than they needed to, it brought me great freedom. If they had actually eaten the heaping pile of mashed potatoes and giant piece of steak I was feeding them, they would have been super-sized children!

I used to prepare their plates with the same portion sizes I gave myself: a large dinner plate with a large serving of potatoes, meat and two veggies. I was always discouraged when they would say they were finished and it looked as if their plates had not been touched. The truth was that my kids were eating but I was giving them so much food that you couldn't tell they had touched anything. I felt defeated thinking my kids were not good eaters, and they felt equally defeated because they were always being hounded to eat more! When I learned about portion sizes, it entirely changed the climate from defeat to victory at our dinner table.

The Kid Friendly ADHD and Autism Cookbook explains portion sizes for children. For example, for the average 4-8 year old child:

A serving size of animal protein would be 12 grams, which is about the size of the palm of their hand. If you look at the palm of a four-year-old, that's not much meat.

A serving size for vegetable protein, which is defined as beans, nuts, and seeds, is about a rounded palm full, ¼ cup or the size of a golf ball. That's not much!

Serving sizes of vegetables, fruits and grains:

- Raw leafy vegetables: 1 cup, which equals about one large leaf of romaine lettuce.
- Fruit: 1 medium
- Pasta, rice, cooked cereal: ½ cup
- Potato: 1 medium

I began giving my children small portions on a salad-size plate. When I put half of a large baked potato, a golf-ball-sized scoop of beans, and a piece of meat the size of their palm on their plate, within two bites you could actually tell they had eaten! They began to ask for "seconds" because they actually would finish their meat and desire more. I felt victorious because my kids were eating and they felt great because I was no longer bugging them to eat more.

Kids will often eat what their bodies need. Therefore, if you give your child a palm-sized piece of meat and they ask for more, make sure to give them more. Don't think, "Oh, they've had their serving of meat, they're done." As children grow, there are times they need more than the recommended amount.

My pediatrician told me that toddlers have a 48-hour eating cycle. That's why many times when you sit down at the dinner table they just pick at their food. She said that toddlers usually eat one good meal every 48 hours. Keep that in mind and make sure all your snacks for your toddler are full of nutrients and good living foods. Sometimes those snack times end up being that "one" meal! So, don't be offended if your toddler sits down and only picks at their food – it's totally normal. Just keep giving them small portions and they will grow into a normal eating cycle!

Chapter 10

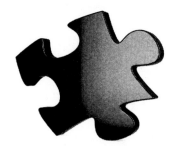

MENU PLANNING:
The Key to Victory

I'm now going to walk you through a process that will guarantee success. It does take a bit to set it up but, once you do, it will only take you moments each week to create a healthy meal plan for your family!

When I first began our healthy eating plan, everything was homemade, requiring many individual ingredients, so I spent hours trying to figure out a system to keep me from running to the grocery store multiple times per day. I finally figured out a menu planning system that made our lives sane again! It also helped create a budget, which made eating this way much more affordable. Many have shared that this menu planning system is the one thing that has really helped them stay on track with healthy eating. I pray this tool helps you as much as it did me!

Here are the eight steps to menu planning:

1. Choose Your Plan
2. Add Your Activities

3. Create Your Plan
4. Make a Shopping List
5. Make a Shopping Plan
6. Shop
7. Time Saving Food Preparation for the Week
8. Celebrate!

Now let's look at this step-by-step process in detail.

CHOOSE YOUR PLAN

The first step is to select a meal-planning guide sheet that will best suit your needs. Read through the following four guides and select the one that stands out to you as "do-able." If you're more visual, like I am, you may want to turn toward the back of the book and look at the meal ideas. This may help you to decide which guide will be easiest for you to use.

MEAL PLANNING GUIDE 1: This menu is totally complete for you. The grocery list is included: you just need to alter it to what you already have in your house. All you need to do to implement this list is go shopping and get cookin'.

MEAL PLANNING GUIDE 2: This menu is completed for you with the exception of dinners. It also has a shopping list included. You can fill in the dinners of your choice from the dinner section of the cookbook. Look up the recipes and add to the shopping list what you need for dinner.

MEAL PLANNING GUIDE 3: This menu allows you to fill in breakfast, lunch, and dinner for your family. Use the idea sections to generate ideas for meals and then look up the recipes to create a shopping list.

MEAL PLANNING GUIDE 4: This is a blank menu for you to fill out to meet the needs and tastes of your family. Select meals and snacks, look up recipes and create your shopping list.

After selecting a meal planning sheet, make numerous copies of it and keep them in a folder or bin in your kitchen for quick access in the future.

MENU PLANNING

QUICK TIP #1:
Be prepared! Having many guides copied and ready to go will help you succeed. What busy mom has time to run to the copier each week?

QUICK TIP #2:
Take a little extra time and create a sound plan from the beginning!

I began with the blank meal-planning guide. It took extra time when I first sat down and planned breakfast, lunch and snacks for my family, tailoring it to our dietary needs and tastes.

On my computer I then created a shopping list for the breakfast, lunch and snack part of my menu, which remain the same week after week. I then post the shopping list on my fridge and highlight items as I run out of them.

I left the dinner part of the planning sheet blank and then made multiple copies. Now, each week I only need to fill in dinners and I leave the rest of the plan as is.

After planning my dinners, I add to the shopping list on the fridge additional items I will need for dinners. If I notice that my kids quit eating a breakfast (for example: oatmeal), I remove that breakfast and put in a new one. Same with lunch or snacks – if my kids quit eating them, I just switch out that item for a new item. This helps keep my meal planning easy and they actually eat what they are given to eat. Since my menu and shopping list are stable (other than dinners), it makes it easy to budget and keeps meals nutritious and varied.

I've been using this system for over four years and it works great! Once you get it set up, it only takes about 10 minutes a week to plop in dinners, make any switches needed and add dinner ingredients to your shopping list. I plan meals for two weeks but I shop weekly. One week I buy all I can that is non-perishable and the second week I just pick up replacement produce.

ADD YOUR ACTIVITIES

Now that you've selected a meal-planning guide, get out your calendar and look at your schedule of events. Before you plan your meals, write on your meal plan the nights you have events going on. This is a critical step!

CREATE YOUR PLAN

Using your meal-planning guide, go to the meal ideas section of this book and plan all the meals that you will need for the week. At this time don't worry about a shopping list – just fill in the meals you'll be preparing. For nights with scheduled events make sure to select a crock-pot or frozen meal idea.

The next step is to look up the recipes for your meal plan and create a shopping list.

QUICK TIP #3:
Have a stable breakfast, lunch, snack menu and shopping list. Print it out and keep it on your fridge so each week you just add dinner ingredients. This saves time and energy, and makes it easy to budget.

MAKE A SHOPPING PLAN

Now that your shopping list is complete, the next step is to come up with a shopping plan. Look at the foods you need and the best place to get them. Often, people go to the grocery store plus a whole-sale store such as Costco or Sam's Club. Take a look at your list, decide where you need to go, and devise an efficient route to get all you need.

My route is a bit more drastic then the mainstream person because I am shopping for six people on a gluten-free, dairy-free, sugar-free diet – so I make a few more stops than you probably will have to make. But I start off the day with my favorite coffee, put my music in the CD player and enjoy a few hours of time out! I go in the store, buy what I need and go to the next stop. Stick to your list and don't wander in the stores – it will save you time and help you stick to your budget. These few hours spent keep our family prepared and flowing smoothly for the week.

There are times when I have to take my children shopping with me – all four of them, ages 11, 7, 5, and 3. We actually have a great time together, though it's not quite as efficient. I do have to just have the mindset that it will take a while – this makes it enjoyable for me.

I give the kids items that they have to search for as we go along. Once they find their item and place it in the cart, I give them a new item to look for. This keeps them busy and focused as we shop. The other thing is that we are always on the lookout for something new! So, they have their eyes peeled for the new item we get to try.

Quick Tip #4:
Doing all the shopping and prep work on the same day saves time and money. I find that when I do take a chunk of time on Saturdays and get the shopping and prep work done, we do not run to the store during the week and I always have what I need.

Time Saving Food Preparation for the Week

Now that you've brought everything home, the last step is to get it ready for the week. You'll want to clean all the fruits and vegetables that you can. This is what I do.

Vegetables & Fruit

Lettuce (Romaine or Leafy Lettuce): Cut off the end and wash each leaf. Roll out three paper towels and lay one layer of leaves on the paper towels, then put three more paper towels on top and continue to layer until all the leaves are gone. Then, roll up the lettuce and place it in a large Ziploc bag. The bag does not usually seal and that's okay. The lettuce will last for at least one week.

BROCCOLI/CAULIFLOWER: Remove flowerets, wash thoroughly, pat dry and place in a large Ziploc bag with a piece of paper towel. They will keep for about one week.

CELERY: Chop into lengths, wash and put in a Ziploc bag.

CARROTS: Don't clean these ahead of time because they dry out quickly. I buy a bag of large carrots and when we eat them, I wash them and cut off each end. Don't peel them since that's where the nutrition is (if they're not organic, you *do* want to peel them due to pesticides). My kids love to eat the big carrots. My son at four years old would eat an entire large carrot.

APPLES, PEARS, PLUMS, GRAPES, BLUEBERRIES AND CHER-RIES: Wash and pat these fruits dry. I have them available for my kids to grab out of the fridge and eat at anytime.

QUICK TIP #5:

By prepping, all the fruits and vegetables are ready to go. I can reach in the fridge anytime for a healthy, quick snack.

By taking the time to prepare fruits and vegetables this way, I don't end up throwing them away. If I don't clean the broccoli and cauliflower, it ends up in the garbage because I never have time to clean it once the week begins. By having the fruits clean, the kids can just grab them and go.

I know fruits and vegetables lose some nutrients when you cut them, however, if I don't cut them – we don't eat them.

While storing in Ziplocs is not the healthiest option, it is the most convenient. If you have enough glass containers, use those over the Ziplocs!

Freezer & Crock-Pot Meals

Saturday is the time that I prepare any meals I need to make ahead of time. If we have three nights of activities, I will either plan crock-pot meals or I may make some taco meat, chili, and lasagna and put them in the freezer for those nights. Then all I have to do is take out taco meat, toss out the veggies and some fruit and we have a healthy dinner in minutes.

Quick Tip #6:

Double it! If I'm making chili, tacos, sloppy joes, soup, or anything that I can double, I fix a double or triple batch and freeze it. Then I not only have a meal for later in the week but future meals as well. I keep a list on the freezer of what I put in there. Then, if I do get stuck one night and need a quick meal, I can look at my list and pull something out. You will find the freezer list in the back of the book as well. Copy it and use it for being extra prepared!

Celebrate!

You did it! It was a lot of work but you've now set up your own family-tailored meal-planning system. You're ready to feed your family a healthy diet for an entire week. Have a blessed week not going to the store every day or wondering, "What should I make for dinner tonight?" Enjoy the benefits of all your diligence and preparation! As you continue, it will get faster and easier.

Chapter 11

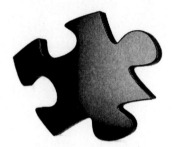

HELPING THE KIDS ADJUST

The first step is to determine what you do and do not want your children to eat – then get everything you don't want them eating out of the house. I suggest that as you run out of food items that you don't want your kids eating any longer, replace them with a similar, healthy alternative. For example: If your kids really love microwave popcorn, eat up what you have and, when you run out, buy some coconut oil, grass-fed or organic butter, sea salt and uncooked popcorn. Then, instead of using the microwave, just melt some coconut oil in a pan and pop the popcorn in that. Drizzle some butter over it and top it off with sea salt – you have a healthy alternative!

If you work and you need popcorn for your child's afternoon snack, pop it in the morning as you cook breakfast and store it in a paper bag or glass container until after school.

Don't try to go cold turkey with everything in your house – it won't go over well. If you make the process slow and easy, it will stick, and your kids will transition more easily.

Some children are a little more choosy than others about their food, while others actually have sensory issues where the texture, smell, strong taste, or lack of taste makes foods seem impossible to eat. Food therapy is available for children with those food issues.

I have a little box of tricks that our family developed as we began exploring new foods. Above all, make eating and meal times *fun*.

As a family we focus on fun and bonding, not the food, at mealtime. Every night we have each person share his or her best part of the day. By the time all six of us have shared and commented on each other's day, twenty minutes or so has gone by and dinner is over. We try to keep the focus off the food, but if food does come up, here are some things that we've done to encourage our kids to eat up!

SAFE MEALTIMES

Begin changing the atmosphere at mealtime. Make this time a relaxed, non-stressful time to connect with each other. Discuss highlights and lows of the day. Use this time to help (especially those "tweeners") process those low times they are experiencing. Meals are a time that my kids are really open to discussion. I think it's because it's an intimate and safe setting. We often use this as a time to pray for friends who are not being kind or have hurt them throughout the day.

Make sure to daily eat at least one meal together as a family. There is so much amazing research on the benefits of a family that eats together. I suggest you look into it if you don't already know about it.

PLAY WITH YOUR FOOD

Kids must touch their food! This may require you to make a major mind shift, but it's an important developmental process for your children. Touching food is an extremely important part of developing a varied pallet. That's why there is a "finger food" stage for the little ones. It exposes them to new textures, smells, colors, shapes, and tastes. Squeezing the peas, smearing the mashed potatoes all over their tray, and licking the banana goo off their finger is a critical part of developing a less picky eater in the future.

I learned this when my oldest was six. She was my "neat chick." She never really liked a finger food unless it was clean, so she didn't do much with exploring foods. My second, however, explored a bit more and is much less picky. I had this information when my last two children were young and, wow, they really explored their food! I can truly say that I have not found a food they will not eat!

So, let your kids play with their food, it will help them become great eaters in the future. We actually build sculptures when we have mashed potatoes; the kids build and share their creations with the family. They get pretty creative!

We've taught them that when we're at grandma and grandpa's house, we don't build with food. We've never had an issue with inappropriate mashed potato sculptures at Thanksgiving dinner!

I'VE SEEN THAT BEFORE!

Children need to *see* new foods. This means they have to have multiple exposures to new foods. Most of the research points to about 10-20 times before they will actually eat it. However, if you have a child with sensory issues or a picky eater (start declaring over your child "You are a great eater!" and see what happens) they may need to see it more like 50-100 times – I say this from personal experience.

On my oldest daughter's plate, I began by just putting a potato on the plate, then I had her touch it, and then taste it – just one taste. (When you're doing this, use a piece of a potato to make it less overwhelming to them). Finally, one day she took a taste and the next thing I knew, the potato was gone! We're now doing the same thing with my second daughter and squash. So, don't give up, just keep presenting it to them, and *be patient*.

"NO, THANK YOU" HELPING

Set up your child's plate with a little bit of everything on it. They have to taste everything on their plate but if they don't like an item, they can say, "No, thank you." If they say, "No, thank you" to the entire plate, I allow my children to make a peanut butter or sun butter sandwich – but they must do it alone. I make it very clear that I have already made dinner and they will have to make and clean up if they so choose to make a sandwich. So, from age five on, my daughter has done this. She will get out the bread, peanut butter and honey, make her sandwich, put everything away and rejoin us at the table where we will finish dinner together.

When she was almost eleven, I made a meal she really didn't like so she decided to make a sandwich. Then it was a trickle down effect; my second daughter chimed in, "I want a sandwich." (You know how it is – when the oldest does something, everyone follows suit.) I said, "No problem, Hannah is making the second dinner tonight, just give her your order." Then the boys followed right behind. I sat delighted, as my ten-year-old made four sandwiches and served her sister and brothers. She sat down and said, "Wow, that was a lot of work." Needless to say, she has never done that again!

At the beginning of the "No, thank you" helping we just had them taste each item on their plate one time. But as they got more used to the new way we were eating, we increased it to three tastes of each item before they could make a sandwich.

Remember to give them very small portions of foods they don't love yet, because there will be a day when they take three tastes, the serving will be gone and they will ask for more. After we switched to tasting each food three times, our dinner table became a baseball field!

Yes, baseball. Each night when we sat down, the kids would eat something and go, "Strike one, strike two, strike three," then they would yell, "You're out" and we would all laugh. Occasionally, a food would strike out but this, too, became less and less. By the time we were doing baseball, most meals did not strike out – just a food item here and there.

DIP!

Dip, dip, dip is the next tip. If the kids can dip they will be much more apt to eat it. So, find some good dips. Ketchup is one many use, but make sure it's free from corn syrup; fruit juice sweetened ketchup is best.

There is a veggie dip in the recipe section of this book that works great for any kind of vegetable. Organic ranch and Italian dressings are good in moderation. Make sure they're organic because conventional dressings contain MSG, preservatives, corn syrup, antibiotics, and hormones to name a few.

My youngest was allergic to everything when he was little (now he can eat everything). He reacted to almost every food we gave him but, being a little guy, he wanted to dip like everyone else. So, I gave him a dipping bowl with water in it and he was happy as a clam, dipping away. When he realized it was different from everyone else's, I colored it with juices like beet juice.

FIRST RESPONSE IS ALWAYS "NO!"

Some children (and adults) will react to any change, even a good change with, "No!" The reason for this is that they need time to process the change. Once they have some time, they're okay with it.

I discovered this with my daughter. She would wake up and I would say, "We're having pancakes this morning." She would look at me and say, "I hate pancakes." I knew this wasn't true; she loved them. But this happened morning after morning. Then it dawned on me that it didn't matter what I gave her for breakfast, she was actually adjusting to the change from sleep to awake. While that was happening, her first reaction to whatever I gave her for breakfast was, "I hate that. No, I'm not going to eat it!"

One morning, I was trying to get some breakfast in her before she was off to school for the day. She was sitting at the table with sausage, a banana chocolate chip muffin and fruit in front of her. She was crying because she hated what I had made, which, by the way, was her ultimate favorite. I finally took her on my lap and snuggled her, then I explained that her first reaction to whatever was for breakfast was, "No, ick." I told her that she was in control of her body and her body was not in control of her. I said, "You take control. You tell your body that you love these muffins and sausage and then let's take three bites. We will see if your tongue changes its mind as you taste your muffin."

She agreed and said out loud, "No, I like muffins," and took one bite. I asked how it was and she said, "Icky." When she took the second bite, she said, "It's okay." After the third bite she said, "I love these muffins!" I said, "You see, your tongue changed its mind! It really does love the muffins – it must have forgotten."

That's where "your tongue might change its mind" came from. Whenever the kids eat something and say "Ick," we say, "Try again. Maybe your tongue changed its mind." This works great when they say, "I didn't like this the last time you made it." Your response can be a light and fun, "Well, let's see if your tongue changed its mind" and as they acquire new tastes, it actually will!

Explaining to my daughter how her body responds and how to take charge of it to give her time to adjust has actually transferred into other areas of life as well.

HAVE A FAVORITE HANDY

As you begin presenting new food items in your meals, make sure to make one thing that you know your child will eat. For example, whenever I try a new recipe on them, I always make their favorite salad: a basic lettuce salad with purple onion, kalamata olives, goat cheese, pepperoncini peppers, and their favorite Italian dressing. Then, if they don't care for the new recipe, they will be able to fill up on salad.

Little Cooks Make Happy Eaters

One of the best things you can do is to get them cooking! Little chefs will eat their creations and convince everyone else to eat, too. Right now, as I write, my eleven-year-old and her girlfriend are making cookies. We're out of the flour they need so she's experimenting with the flour we do have. No matter what happens, it's great that she's developing a love for cooking good, healthy and creative food!

Presentation

When you're presenting a meal, have a variety of textures and make it colorful with various tastes. Believe it or not, they will eat more on a colorful plate. I know when I heard this I thought, "I barely have time to make dinner let alone think about if it's pretty." But with menu planning, it's very easy – you have everything at your fingertips.

So, for a colorful lunch, let's say I'm making pesto pasta (green); I toss on some carrots (yellow), an apple (red), and a glass of water – quick, easy and appealing to the eye. The meal has various tastes, colors, and textures!

I usually spring new snack foods or meals on my children when they have friends over. This has proven to be an excellent way to get my kids to try new stuff. I've developed a reputation as the house where you never know what you'll be served, but the guests love it. My good friend's daughter was having a sleepover at our house and I pulled out some blood oranges for a snack. She looked at me puzzled and said, "You just never know what you're going to get to eat at the Schulte's house." By the way, she loved the blood oranges!

Funny food names help kids eat food they normally wouldn't. At our house, cashews are moon rocks and macadamia nuts are baseballs. One day in the car, my kids were asking for a snack. Not thinking, I replied with, "I have cashews." They all said, "No way!" Then I said, "I mean moon rocks," and they all replied, "Oh, okay."

Educate

Learning about what they are eating has really helped my kids stick to eating the way we do. I teach them what we are eating and why, as well as what we are *not* eating and why.

One day, my three-year-old son was sitting next to his grand-father having some cereal. My son asked, "Is that cow's milk?" My father-in-law answered, "Why, yes it is." My son then began, "Do you know what they do with cow's milk?" I quickly cut him off before he went into a sermon on the subject. I told him we respect what others choose to eat; it was okay for grandpa – just not for us. This is a key to kids *wanting* to eat healthy, not just because mom says so.

Eating Vegetables

Vegetables, the dreaded vegetables! How do we get our kids to eat these essentials? This "no-brainer" took me forever to figure out and it's so simple: switch up your cooking methods.

My kids wouldn't eat green beans. I'd buy frozen green beans and boil them until they were soggy (just like my mom did) and my kids refused them time after time. I was discussing this with a friend and she suggested that I sauté them in olive oil with a bit of garlic salt. I tried it – they were wonderful and my kids ate up the entire batch.

I then purchased my favorite cookbook, *Asparagus to Zucchini*, which teaches how to prepare and store various vegetables. It's like *gold*! Every time my kids don't like a vegetable, I simply whip out my book and try a different way to cook it. Or, if they quit eating a veggie, I will pull out this awesome cookbook and find a new recipe to get them eating that veggie again. So, if you're stuck, remember: you can boil, sauté, grill, raw, broil or stir-fry them up!

Camouflage

Another idea, a bit more time-consuming, is to hide the good stuff. Puree vegetables like carrots, onion, broccoli and cauliflower to put in chili, meatloaf, taco meat, or spaghetti sauce. Or, hide spinach, avocado, and beets in a darn good smoothie. You can also put beans and spinach into cookies and brownies – they taste great.

There are a few cookbooks that devote themselves exclusively to this method of cooking and they're fun to play around with – not super healthy but a great place to start. I have one called *The Sneaky Chef* that I use as a starting point, and then I modify the recipes to fit our diet, making them a bit healthier here and there.

Soups are another place to hide vegetables – just make sure not to use their real name. One of the soups my kids love, we call "Mexisoup." If they knew it was really called "egg-plant tomato soup," I have a feeling they might run the other way. A good way to start your kids on soups, if they're not used to them, is to give them something to dip into the soup, like a grilled cheese sandwich or organic corn chips!

Viking Cauliflower

You can also try vegetables in different colors. My daughter loves cauliflower, so one day I brought home the yellow variety. She was adamant that she wasn't going to eat it. I told her it would taste just like the white, so she finally ventured a bite. To her surprise, it did! Voila, success with a new food! The next week I came home with a purple cauliflower and she dug right in, creatively suggesting we serve purple and yellow cauliflower at a Vikings football party!

We tried different colors with watermelon, carrots, and potatoes. She was very successful at trying these new things and she became more adventurous with new foods because she'd experienced success.

Sitting at the Table

I'm often asked, "How do you get your kids to sit at the table?" It took some time for this one to develop. We never had that much success until we started occupational therapy. The tips we learned would work for every child, not just those with sensory issues.

We used an exercise ball at the dinner table – we removed our daughter's chair and gave her the ball to sit on; she sat easily at the table for 15 minutes. We then moved from a ball at the table to a little pad with bumps and ridges that we set on her chair. When she then sat on that, we were able to reach our goal of 20 minutes for dinner.

We used consequences if they didn't sit at the table until a timer went off. We started at five minutes and continued to increase the time, bit by bit. We now sit at the dinner table and enjoy each other. But with each one of our little ones, there was a time of training – it's a learned skill. My youngest child so loves people that he has never had a problem sitting at the table. Each child is different and I hope these tips help you make dinnertime a fun and enjoyable family time. The more relaxed your dinnertime is, the more your kids will eat!

Making It Stick

After all is said and done, the biggest thing that will help you be successful is to take baby steps. Look at it as a lifestyle change, not a diet. When Lilli, my second daughter, asked me, "Mom, when are we going to be done with this diet?" I looked at her and responded, "Never." I realized that our lives had changed forever and we would never go back to eating the way we used to. We will forever be changed.

You know yourself and how much you can handle. Pick one thing, and once you have a handle on that, go to the next thing. Make sure to engage someone in the process with you to keep you motivated and accountable. Write your goals down and display them to keep you inspired. Remember, you're building the health of your children for now and the rest of their lives. The tastes they develop under your roof will stick with them their entire lives.

Give yourself time and grace. I've heard that it takes six to eight weeks for a new habit to replace an old. If you make a mistake, it's okay! Forgive yourself and move on – keep going, don't give up. I know you can do it!

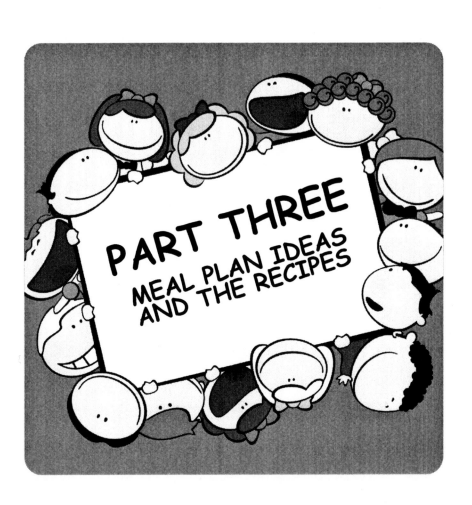

PART THREE
MEAL PLAN IDEAS
AND THE RECIPES

Chapter 12

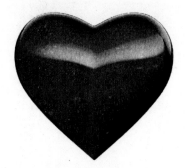

MEAL PLAN IDEAS

T he meal ideas and recipes are kid tested and approved by my "picky" eater. It took a full year to get her to eat a potato and she now will eat everything in this book! It's my hope that your children will enjoy these meals that are fun, nutritious, unique, and delicious.

WHAT YOU NEED TO KNOW – DAIRY

In this book I use mainly a mix of goat and sheep cheese. I do not use any cow-based dairy. If you must be on a 100% dairy-free diet, use a rice, nut or soy-based cheese of the same variety in the same proportion. Local co-ops will have mozzarella and cheddar varieties. If you're able to use goat or sheep cheese, I suggest that you use goat Gouda, goat cheddar, or goat mozzarella in place of the rice or soy mozzarella and cheddar. It has more flavor and melts much better. You can also use Pecorino Romano cheese for Parmesan; just check the packaging to make sure it's from sheep.

Try grass-fed butter – it's so pure that many people with dairy issues can eat it. But if that doesn't work for you, use Earth Balance sticks, in equal portions, in place of the butter. My family is highly sensitive to cow's milk dairy but we are able to do grass-fed butter, sheep and goat cheese.

GLUTEN OR NO GLUTEN

If you're on a gluten-free diet, these recipes are ready to go for you. If you are able to eat gluten, you can use whole wheat flour with these recipes in equal proportion. With the use of whole wheat flour, you will get a denser variety of the item you're baking. Try some of the gluten-free (GF) flours; they're fun and it's good to mix it up a bit.

WHERE TO FIND IT?

In the recipes, I list some brand names as well as some food items that may not be common. You will be able to find most of these at your local co-op. I haven't had any problem finding them at co-ops when we travel all over the U.S. You can also find them on various websites by just doing a search for the product you would like. Or look for these items at Trader Joe's – they tend to be cheaper.

FOR BREAKFAST

PANCAKES

*(I have found these very hard to make well homemade.
I use the Kinnikinnick Foods brand.)*

◆Oatmeal Pancakes　　　　　　　◆Gingerbread Pancakes

◆Puff Pancake

OATMEAL (STEEL-CUT OATS)

Topping suggestions

◆Grass-fed butter,　　　　　　　◆Almond milk,
honey, Cinnamon　　　　　　　　　agave nectar

◆Fresh or frozen fruit

MUFFINS

◆Banana Chocolate Chip　　　　　　　　　◆Blueberry

◆Berry Yummy　　　　　　　◆Veggie Surprise

QUICK BREADS

◆Zucchini　　　◆Banana

CARAMEL ROLLS

CINNAMON ROLLS

FRENCH TOAST WITH A SIDE OF FRESH FRUIT

BAKED BLUEBERRY-STUFFED FRENCH TOAST

Topping suggestions:

- Agave nectar
- Honey
- Grass-fed butter
- Pure maple syrup

EGG MUFFINS

- Mexican
- Italian

JAPANESE BREAKFAST

ENGLISH BREAKFAST

EGG BAKE

BREADLESS EGG BAKE

OMELETS

GROUND TURKEY SAUSAGE
w/GF toast, bagels or English muffins

LEFTOVER DINNER
(My kids love leftovers for breakfast!)

IDEAS WITHOUT RECIPES

TURKEY BACON
(nitrite/sulfite free)

Served with your favorite fresh fruit and GF toast topped with your choice of organic peanut butter, fruit juice-sweetened jelly, or honey.

GF (GLUTEN FREE) BAGELS/ENGLISH MUFFINS
Kinnikinnick Foods brand is tasty!

Topping suggestions:

+ *Tofutti* cream cheese
+ *Tofutti* cream cheese & sliced fruit
+ Nut butter (peanut, sunflower, almond, etc.) w/fruit
+ Juice-sweetened jelly, honey or agave nectar

GF (GLUTEN FREE) CEREAL
w/rice milk or almond milk & fresh fruit

CORN FLAKES
Nature's Path — fruit juice-sweetened

ORGANIC CORN FLAKES

GLUTEN FREE GRANOLA

BLUEBERRY OR PLAIN GLUTEN-FREE WAFFLES

(Van's Natural Foods is a good brand)

Topping suggestions:

- Fresh or frozen fruit
- Agave Nectar
- Fruit juice-sweetened jelly

- Honey
- Grass-fed butter
- Pure maple syrup (no sugar added)

ORGANIC EGGS & TURKEY BACON

(nitrite/sulfite-free)

w/organic hash brown potatoes
(there are frozen varieties)

fresh fruit & GF toast

HOMEMADE HASH BROWNS

(or use frozen organic hash browns)

w/whole wheat toast & fresh fruit

OR

w/turkey bacon or sausage
(nitrite-free)

FOR LUNCH

Every lunch is served with a raw vegetable with or without dip. I rotate the vegetables with the days (and seasons): cauliflower, broccoli, carrots, celery, green beans, pea pods, tomatoes, etc. I serve fruit for dessert each day.

RICE AND BEANS

Serve w/organic sour cream, organic corn chips

PESTO PASTA

CILANTRO PESTO PASTA

TUNA SANDWICH

TUNA AND CRACKERS

TUNA MELTS

BUILD-A-SUB

BUILD YOUR OWN SALAD

QUESADILLAS

w/goat Gouda, rice or soy cheese, refried or black beans, salsa, beef/chicken, any other toppings of your choice

EGG SALAD SANDWICH

TACOS IN A BAG

ORGANIC PEANUT BUTTER & JELLY TORTILLAS
(or sunbutter)

GF NOODLES W/OLIVE OIL
& PECORINO CHEESE

MAC-N-CHEESE

ORGANIC RED PEPPER &TURKEY ROLL UPS

PIZZA PARTY

INCREDIBLE PIZZA TORTILLAS

FRIED EGG SANDWICH

GF ENGLISH MUFFIN PIZZAS

PIZZA BOATS

ITALIAN DIPPERS

FRITTATAS

JEANNIE'S PEANUT DIP OVER GF NOODLES

PIZZA PACKS

IDEAS WITHOUT RECIPES

SPAGHETTI w/BROWN RICE NOODLES

LETTUCE SALAD w/CUBED MEAT FOR PROTEIN
(chicken, turkey, etc.)

Topper ideas:

- Grape tomatoes
- Grated carrots
- Kalamata olives
- Cucumbers

SANDWICHES & WRAPS
(GF bread or ivory teff tortillas)

- Turkey • Beef • Chicken

SOUP & GRILLED GOAT GOUDA SANDWICHES ON GF BREAD
(There are many good organic soups at co-ops and grocery stores.)

MEAT (DELI STYLE)
GOAT CHEESE (GOUDA, HERBED)
w/rice or soy crackers

SALAMI
on GF bread, w/mustard

ORGANIC CORN-ON-THE-COB & DELI TURKEY
(Rolled up for finger food)

CHILI

w/corn bread or GF breadsticks

(Chili can be leftover or frozen, reheated, and sent to school in a heated thermos.)

◆ *ALL MEATS SHOULD BE NITRITE FREE.*

FOR DINNER

CHILI #1 OR FRESH VEGGIE CHILI

w/corn bread

CHILI #2

w/corn bread & maple butter

HAMBURGER SOUP

TOMATO BASIL WILD-CAUGHT SALMON

BROILED OR GRILLED WILD-CAUGHT SALMON

STIR-FRY

w/brown rice & fruit

HOMEMADE PIZZA

BURRITO BOWLS

w/chips, salsa, guacamole & fruit

BBQ Ribs

w/organic corn-on-the-cob,
mashed potatoes, broccoli & salad

Cheryl's Done-at-Noon Stew

Enchilada Soup in the Crock-Pot

w/tortilla chips, Tofutti sour cream & fruit

Chinese Roast in the Crock-Pot

w/brown rice, asparagus, salad & fruit

Brisket in the Crock-Pot

w/baked potatoes and carrots, peas, salad & fruit

Beef, Tomato & Noodle Hot Dish

w/GF dinner rolls, peas & fruit

Beef Roast

w/vegetables, salad & fruit

Roast Chicken

w/vegetables

Hamburger Hot Dish

w/GF dinner rolls, salad & fruit

French Dip Sandwiches

w/raw veggies & dip, fruit & sweet potato chips

SPICY FRENCH DIP SANDWICHES

ASPARAGUS SOUP
w/GRILLED GOAT CHEESE SANDWICHES

CHICKEN & BROWN RICE SOUP

EGGPLANT TOMATO SOUP
w/GRILLED GOAT GOUDA SANDWICHES

WINTER ROOT SOUP
w/GRILLED GOAT CHEESE SANDWICHES

QUINOA & BLACK BEANS
w/artichokes, salad & fruit

THAI CHICKEN SATAY
w/brown rice, salad & fried wontons

TOMATO BASIL TART
w/salad, fruit & asparagus

LITTLE CHEDDAR MEAT LOAVES
w/mashed potatoes, peas & salad

OVEN ROASTED DIJON CHICKEN
w/mashed potatoes, artichokes & salad

SWEET & SOUR CHICKEN
w/brown rice & broccoli

Stir-Fried Steak & Rice

Grilled Flank Steak

Teriyaki Meat Marinade

Dairy Free Stuffed Jumbo Shells

Black Bean Stew

Homemade Loaded Spaghetti Sauce
w/pasta or dipper sandwiches

Spaghetti and Meatballs
w/garlic toast & salad

Baked Spaghetti
w/garlic toast & salad

Baked Ziti
w/garlic toast & salad

Jeanne's Peanut Dip over Pasta, Raw Snap Peas & Raw Red Pepper Strips

Jeanne's Ratatouille

Curried Chicken & Brown Rice
Grilled Sirloin Steak
w/artichokes, baked or mashed potatoes, salad & fruit

ENCHILADAS

SPINACH & ROASTED RED PEPPER ENCHILADAS

SWEET & SPICY CHICKEN STRIPS

HIDDEN VEGGIE LASAGNA

LINGUINE
w/roasted red peppers, peas & pine nuts

CROCK-POT DILL ROAST w/CREAMY GRAVY

CROCK-POT CHICKEN w/POTATOES

BUFFALO CHICKEN WINGS (DRUMMIES)

ASIAN CHICKEN WINGS (DRUMMIES)

SESAME CHICKEN STRIPS

IDEAS WITHOUT RECIPES

GRILLED CHICKEN BREAST

w/mashed orange potatoes, asparagus & salad

TACOS

(Use your favorite taco seasoning and meat)

w/beans, chips & guacamole

TACO SALAD

(Use corn chips crushed on bottom for base)

w/chips & guacamole

BURGERS

(1/2 Buffalo, 1/2 Grass-fed Beef)

w/GF buns, sweet potato fries, salad & fruit

CAMPFIRE MEAL

GF Brats/Hot Dogs (nitrite-free)

w/veggie chips, veggies & dip, & fruit

BROILED STEAK

w/baked sweet potatoes, artichokes & salad

GRILLED STEAK w/GARLIC BUTTER

w/baked potatoes, broccoli & salad

THE RECIPES

BREAKFAST

In recipes that call for cheese I use goat or sheep cheese, which my family is fine with. If that is not an option for you, I have put 100% dairy-free alternatives in parenthesis.

BAKED BLUEBERRY-STUFFED FRENCH TOAST

1 loaf GF French Bread (or GF bread of choice)

8 oz. Tofutti Cream Cheese

1½ c. Rice Milk

2 c. Blueberries

¼ c. Organic Maple Syrup

8 Organic eggs

¼ c. Melted Earth Balance (EB) or Grass-fed Butter

Preheat oven to 350 degrees. Spray a 9 x 13 pan with olive oil spray. Cut bread into one-inch cubes and place half of them in the pan as the bottom layer. Cut the cream cheese into cubes and sprinkle over the bread. Layer one cup of blueberries next. Then sprinkle the remaining bread cubes over the existing layers. Add the last cup of blueberries over the top. Break the eggs into a bowl and whisk briskly. In a separate bowl, combine rice milk, syrup, and melted EB. Pour mixture over dry ingredients in pan. Try to saturate all the bread. Place pan in oven and bake for about one hour until toothpick inserted comes out clean and top is golden brown.

Oatmeal Pancakes

1 c. GF Oats	½ c. Potato Flour
½ c. Tapioca Flour	½ c. Corn Flour (or meal)
2½ tsp. Baking Powder	1 tsp. Sea Salt
2 Organic Eggs	2 c. Rice Milk
2 T. Brown Sugar	5 T. melted EB or Grass-fed Butter

Grind oats in a blender or food processor until a fine powder. Pour into a large bowl; mix in potato, tapioca, and corn flour along with baking powder and salt. In a medium bowl beat eggs, whisk in milk and brown sugar. Slowly and gently, add liquid ingredients into dry ingredients until well blended. Do not over stir. Let batter sit for several minutes. Heat skillet or griddle to medium high heat (325 degrees), grease. Drop batter by heaping tablespoons and cook until bottoms are golden brown and bubbles are popping on the surface, about 1 minute. Turn and cook 1 minute more. Keep warm.

Serve with fruit-sweetened jam, honey, real maple syrup, or agave nectar (my favorite!)

◆ To decrease glycemic index, I mix maple syrup with agave nectar. This gives a maple syrup taste without the high spike in sugar levels. Play around with it until you find a flavor blend your kids like. I use ½ cup agave with 1 tablespoon maple syrup. Extra can be stored in a sealed container in the fridge.

Gingerbread Pancakes

Step One:

Combine the following dry ingredients in a bowl and mix well.

1 c. Dark Teff Flour   1 c. Tapioca Flour

1 tsp. Gum   1 tsp. Ground Ginger

1 tsp. Baking Soda   ½ tsp. Sea Salt

2 tsp. Baking Powder (Aluminum-Free)

Step Two:

Mix the following in a small bowl.

1 c. Unsweetened Almond Milk (or Rice Milk)

1 T. Organic Lemon Juice

Step Three:

Mix the following wet ingredients in a large mixing bowl.

2 Organic Eggs   ⅓ c. Honey

¼ c. Maple Syrup (or honey)   ⅓ c. Olive Oil

Step Four:

Stir in Almond Milk/Lemon Juice mixture.

Step Five:

Slowly add dry ingredients to wet ingredients and mix with large spoon until smooth.

Step Six:

In a pan or griddle greased with olive oil or grass-fed butter, cook on medium heat for about 5 minutes per side. Top with honey, maple syrup or agave nectar.

Puffed Pancake

1 c. Milk (Rice or Almond)   ¼ tsp. Sea Salt

6 Organic Eggs   1 c. Millet Flour

6 T. EB or Grass-fed Butter

Preheat oven to 450-degrees. Combine milk, salt, eggs, and flour in a blender. Mix on HIGH until blended. In a 9 x 13 pan, melt Earth Balance in the oven, being careful not to burn it. When the butter is melted, remove the pan from the oven, pour pancake mix in HOT pan and quickly put back into the oven. Bake for 20 minutes. Serve HOT with pure maple syrup, fresh fruit, honey, agave, or your favorite topping.

French Toast

3 Organic Eggs   1 c. Almond or Rice Milk

2-3 T. Cinnamon   1 tsp. Vanilla

1 loaf Brown Rice or Millet Bread

Break eggs into a large bowl and whisk well. Add milk and continue to whisk. Sprinkle with cinnamon and add vanilla. (My kids like cinnamon a lot, so I do a thick layer of cinnamon on top of the eggs and then whisk it in.) Dunk bread quickly on both sides in egg mixture and place in greased frying pan or griddle. Flip when golden brown on first side and repeat on second side. Serve with pure maple syrup, honey, agave, or fruit juice-sweetened jelly.

BERRY YUMMY MUFFINS

1 c. Millet Flour	1 c. Brown Rice Flour
1 c. Rice Milk	3 ripe mashed Bananas
¾ c. Honey	½ c. Olive Oil
1 tsp. Sea Salt	2 Organic Eggs
1 tsp. Baking Soda	1 tsp. Baking Powder
¾ c. Blueberries or Cherries	

Preheat oven to 350 degrees. Combine flours, salt, baking soda, baking powder in a bowl. In a separate bowl, mix honey, milk, oil and eggs. Mix mashed bananas into liquid ingredients. Slowly add dry ingredients to wet ingredients and mix well. Fold in berries of choice. Spoon batter, so tins are ½ to ¾ full, into paper lined muffin tins. Place in oven and bake for 20 minutes or until golden brown on top and a toothpick inserted in the center comes out clean. Pop muffins out of the pan and let them cool on a wire rack.

Banana Chocolate Chip Muffins

1 c. Brown Rice Flour	½ c. Tapioca Flour
1 tsp. Baking Soda	½ tsp. Sea Salt
3 ripe mashed Bananas	2 T. Honey
½ c. Maple Syrup or Xylitol	1 Organic Egg
1 tsp. Baking Powder (aluminum-free)	⅓ c. melted EB or Grass-fed Butter
½ c. GF/DF Chocolate Chips	

en to 375 degrees. Line muffin tins. In a large bowl, mix dry ingredients: flours, baking powder, baking soda, and salt. In a separate bowl whip egg, add maple syrup or xylitol/honey, Earth Balance, and bananas, and stir vigorously until well mixed. Slowly add dry ingredients. Fold in chocolate chips. Fill muffin tins ½ to ¾ full and bake for about 20 minutes until toothpick inserted comes out clean. Cool in pan for 5 minutes, then remove and place on a wire rack to cook completely.

◆ Try blueberries instead of chocolate chips for variety.

Blueberry Muffins

1 c. Millet Flour	1 c. Rice Milk
1 c. Brown Rice Flour	1 tsp. Baking Powder
½ c. Honey	½ c. Olive Oil
¼ c. Maple Syrup	1 tsp. Vanilla
1 tsp. Sea Salt	2 Organic Eggs
1 tsp. Baking Soda	¾ c. Blueberries

Preheat oven to 350 degrees. Combine flours, salt, baking soda, baking powder in a bowl. In a separate bowl, mix honey, maple syrup, rice milk, vanilla, oil and eggs. Slowly add dry ingredients to wet ingredients and mix until incorporated. Fold in blueberries. Spoon batter into paper-lined muffin tins, ½ to ¾ full. Place in oven and bake for 20 minutes or until golden brown on top and a toothpick inserted in the center comes out clean. Pop muffins out of the pan and let them cool on a wire rack.

◆Chocolate chips are also tasty in this recipe.

✔ HEAD START TIP: *Muffins and quick breads freeze very well for future quick breakfast foods!*

QUICK BREAD: VEGGIE SURPRISE

½ c. Honey

½ c. Xylitol

½ c. Pure Maple Syrup

1 can Pumpkin

4 Organic Eggs

⅔ c. Earth Balance Sticks

1 shredded Carrot

1 shredded Zucchini

1 T. Golden Ground Flax Seeds

1½ tsp. Sea Salt

1 tsp. Cinnamon

½ tsp. Baking Powder

1 tsp. Ground Cloves

⅔ c. chopped Pecans

2 c. Brown Rice Flour

1½ c. Millet Flour

2 tsp. Baking Soda

Preheat oven to 350 degrees. Grease or line 2 muffin tins. In a large bowl, combine honey, xylitol, maple syrup, Earth Balance and cream until smooth. Stir in pumpkin, zucchini, carrots, and eggs. In a separate bowl, mix together rice and millet flour, baking soda, salt, ground flax, cinnamon, baking powder, and cloves. Fold dry ingredients into creamed ingredients. Stir in pecans. Put into two greased loaf pans. Bake until toothpick inserted into middle comes out clean, about 45 minutes.

◆Muffins can also be made from this batter. Just pour into paper-lined muffin tins and bake until toothpick comes out clear, about 20 minutes.

QUICK BREAD: BANANA

½ c. EB Sticks or Grass-fed Butter

3 Organic Eggs

¼ c. Honey

1¼ c. Millet Flour

½ tsp. Sea Salt

1 tsp. aluminum-free Baking-Powder

¼ c. Maple Syrup

¼ c. Xylitol

3 tsp. Pure Vanilla

1 tsp. Baking Soda

1 c. Brown Rice Flour

3 large mashed *very* ripe Bananas

Preheat oven to 350 degrees. Spray 2 (1.5 qt.) loaf pans with olive oil. Cream the following ingredients together: EB, honey, maple syrup, Xylitol. Add eggs, mashed bananas (peel, place on a plate, and mash with a fork), and vanilla (NOT vanillin), and mix well. In separate bowl mix dry ingredients. Add dry ingredients into wet and mix thoroughly. Pour evenly between the two greased loaf pans. Bake on the center rack for 30-45 minutes (oven temperatures vary), until golden brown and toothpick inserted comes out clean.

QUICK BREAD: ZUCCHINI

3 Organic Eggs

½ c. Olive Oil

½ c. Applesauce

3 tsp. Cinnamon

1 tsp. Sea Salt

1 tsp. Baking Soda

1 tsp. Baking Powder

1 T. Pure Vanilla

¼ c. Corn Flour (meal)	¾ c. Millet Flour
1 c. Brown Rice Flour	2 c. Grated Zucchini
¼ tsp. Cloves	

1 c. Raw Sugar (or ½ c. Maple Syrup & ½ c. Honey)

Combine eggs, oil, applesauce, vanilla and sugar (or honey/maple syrup), and zucchini together. In separate bowl mix flours, spices, baking powder and baking soda. Slowly pour dry ingredients into wet and mix until blended. Pour into 2 (1.5 qt.) loaf pans sprayed with olive oil. Bake at 350 degrees for about 1 hour or until toothpick inserted in center comes out clean.

CARAMEL ROLLS

1 package Bob's Red Mill Wonderful GF Bread Mix

¼ to ½ c. stick of Earth Balance or Grass-fed Butter

2 T. Organic Brown Sugar (*You can also use a mix of ¼ c. honey and ¼ c. maple syrup instead of the sugar – they are equally as tasty!*)

Make bread according to package directions. (It seems overwhelming the first time you do it but don't be discouraged, it gets easier every time.) Place Earth Balance into 9 x 13 glass baking dish. Place in 350-degree oven, melt completely. When melted, remove from oven and sprinkle brown sugar over melted butter, or drizzle maple syrup and honey. Drop spoonfuls of bread dough on top of sugar mixture. Cover with plastic wrap sprayed with olive oil and rise in a warm place for at least 1 hour. Bake according to directions on bread mix package.

CINNAMON ROLLS

1 package Bob's Red Mill
 Wonderful GF Bread Mix

½ c. stick of EB or Grass-
 fed Butter

½ c. Agave Nectar or Honey

3 T. Cinnamon

Make bread according to package directions. (It seems overwhelming the first time you do it but don't be discouraged, it gets easier every time.) Spray a 9 x 13 pan with olive oil, place 1/2 of bread mix in the pan. Wet a spatula and spread dough evenly over bottom of pan. Cut Earth Balance chunks evenly over dough. Sprinkle cinnamon evenly over dough. Drizzle agave or honey over cinnamon. Place the rest of the dough over the cinnamon; again wet the spatula and smooth dough. Cover with plastic wrap sprayed with olive oil and let rise in a warm place for at least 1 hour. Bake according to directions on bread mix package.

GROUND TURKEY SAUSAGE

1 lb. Ground Turkey

1 Organic Egg

1 tsp. Sea Salt

½ tsp. Dried Oregano

¼ tsp. Pepper

1 tsp. Dried Thyme

Put meat in a mixing bowl. Using your hands, work in all the spices and egg. Form the mixture into patties and fry until golden brown on each side in a lightly oiled skillet.

Mexican Egg Muffins

6 Eggs	Salsa (GF)
Sea Salt & Pepper	¼ c. Diced Red Pepper
¼ c. Diced Onion	1 Crushed Clove Garlic
½ cup (or more) Fresh Chopped Cilantro	¼ Cup Shredded Goat Gouda Rice or Soy

Break eggs into a bowl and whisk. Add cilantro, goat cheese (or rice/soy), red pepper, onion, and garlic. Season with salt and pepper and whisk well. Grease 12 muffin tins with oil and fill each muffin tin 1/2 full of egg mixture. Place in preheated 350-degree oven. Bake for 20 minutes. To check if done, insert a toothpick and if it comes out clean the egg muffins are done. Carefully remove each muffin with a fork. Serve with salsa for dipping, or pour over the top.

◆ITALIAN STYLE: use tomato basil goat Gouda (or rice/soy mozzarella) and pecorino (sheep) cheese (if you are able to do cheese other than cow), use Italian parsley instead of cilantro, and serve with pizza or spaghetti sauce for dipping (pages 163 & 183).

English Breakfast

Millet Hot Dog Buns cut into disks	Goat Gouda, Rice or Soy Cheese
Salami – thinly sliced (GF/nitrate-free)	

Slice bread. Place 1 slice of meat and 1 slice of cheese on each piece of bread. Serve open-faced with a side of fresh fruit.

Japanese Breakfast

1½ c. cooked Brown Rice (as directed on package)	1 package Turkey Bacon (nitrate-free)
4 T. Olive Oil	5 Organic Eggs, beaten
½ package Chicken Sausage (GF – nitrate-free)	½ can Unsweetened Pineapple Chunks
1 T. Sea Salt or to taste	3 T. Tamari Soy Sauce
1½ c. chopped Broccoli, Carrots, Celery, & Peas	1 large Onion, diced

✔ Headstart Tip: *Use Organic Frozen Mixed Veggies*

Prepare rice as directed on package. Place bacon in single layer on 9 x 13 pan and put in a preheated 350-degree oven. Cook until crispy (about 20 minutes) and break apart or dice. Dice onion and sauté in olive oil on medium heat until onions are clear. Add eggs and season with salt and pepper. Cook until eggs are fluffy. Remove to a plate. Dice chicken sausage into bite-sized pieces. Place in sauté pan and heat through. Add bacon. Add eggs. Add rice. Add veggies. Cook until heated through. Stir in soy sauce and serve. (*We love to eat this with chopsticks.*)

Oatmeal

Bob's Red Mill GF Oats or any GF Oats	Agave Nectar
Earth Balance or Grass-fed Butter	

Prepare oats according to package. Melt desired amount of Earth Balance. Drizzle with desired amount of agave.

BREADLESS EGG BAKE

6 Eggs

½ Organic Chicken Breakfast
Sausage (GF/nitrate-free)

Sea Salt & Pepper to taste

¾ c. grated Goat Gouda
Cheese (Rice or Soy will
work, too)

Spray 9 x 13 pan with olive oil cooking spray. Preheat oven to 350 degrees. Whisk eggs in small bowl. Add salt, pepper, and cheese. Chop sausage into bite-size pieces and place on bottom of pan. Pour egg mixture over the top and bake for about 20 minutes, until golden brown on top.

EGG BAKE

7 Organic Eggs

1 tsp. Garlic Salt

8oz. Goat Gouda Cheese
(Rice/Soy)

1 loaf Millet or Brown-Rice Bread

2 c. Rice Milk

1 small Onion, diced

1 Package Turkey Bacon
(nitrate-free)

Place bacon in 9 x 13 pan and put it in a 350-degree oven. Bake until crispy. Grease a different 9 x 13 pan. Place half the bread in a layer in the pan. Whisk together eggs and milk. Pour half of the egg mixture over the bread layer. Sprinkle with garlic salt and half each of the bacon, onion, and cheese. Add another layer of bread, then the rest of the egg mixture, and the remainder of the other ingredients. Bake at 350 degrees for about 1 hour or until a toothpick inserted comes out clean.

OMELETTES

6 Organic Eggs   ½ c. Rice Milk

½ c. Goat Gouda Cheese
  or Goat Cheddar (Rice/Soy Cheddar), grated

Place eggs and milk into a bowl and whisk. Place 1 cup of mixture in a skillet sprayed with olive oil or in a griddle. Sprinkle desired amount of cheese on top and allow to cook until egg firms up and cheese melts. Flip ½ of egg on top of itself to make a taco shape – allow to cook for a minute – flip and cook for another minute. Place on a plate and enjoy!

NOTES

LUNCH RECIPES

RICE & BEANS

1 can (15 oz.) Organic Black Beans

2 c. cooked Brown Rice

1 c. Salsa (or to taste)

Tofutti Sour Cream

Organic Corn Chips

Handful Fresh Cilantro, diced

In a large saucepan mix cooked brown rice, black beans, and salsa; heat thoroughly. Serve in a bowl topped with Tofutti sour cream and cilantro. Dip with chips and eat.

EGG SALAD SANDWICH

6 Hard-Boiled Eggs

1 c. or so of Vegenaise Mayo

1 T. diced GF Pickles

1 T. diced Onion (optional)

Peel, dice, and crush hard-boiled eggs in a bowl. Add mayo to taste and texture. Dice onions and celery very fine and mix in. Serve as a sandwich on toasted brown rice/millet or other GF bread, an ivory teff tortilla, GF bagel, or a GF English muffin – Kinnikinnick Foods has a great one.

PESTO

½ c. Olive Oil   ¼ c. Pine Nuts

¼ c. Pecorino Cheese   1 Clove Crushed Garlic

1 large bunch Fresh Basil   1 tsp. Sea Salt

(I usually use one large handful basil with leaves removed from the stems)

In a blender, combine the olive oil (cold or expeller-pressed), pine nuts, pecorino cheese (sheep) or nutritional yeast, & crushed clove of garlic. Puree until smooth. Next add 1 large bunch of fresh basil. Puree until smooth. Next add sea salt to taste. Serve over brown rice pasta, chicken, or rice.

✔ HEAD START TIP: *Pesto freezes well!*

CILANTRO PESTO

4 cloves crushed Garlic   1/3 c. Brazil Nuts

1/3 c. Sunflower Seeds   1/3 c. Pumpkin Seeds

2 c. fresh chopped Cilantro   2 tsp. Dulse Powder

2/3 c. Flaxseed Oil or Olive-   2 T. fresh squeezed Lemon-
   Oil   Juice

Sea Salt to taste

Place oil, nuts and seeds in a blender. Puree until smooth. Add garlic, dulse, and lemon juice; puree. Add cilantro and blend to form a paste. Add sea salt to taste. Serve tossed with brown rice pasta.

TUNA SALAD

2 cans Wild-Caught Tuna   1 c. Veganaise Mayo

Mix Tuna with Mayo to taste.

◆ *To make a sub sandwich, use GF hot dog buns*

SERVING SUGGESTIONS: Put in bowls and dip with crackers. Put on bread, in a pita, or on a wrap. You can add pepperoncini peppers, lettuce, and tomatoes, if desired. We also like it wrapped up in a piece of lettuce. For a tuna melt, assemble salad, put a layer of salad on a slice of GF bread cover it with rice, soy, or goat cheese. Put in a 350-degree oven until cheese is melted and golden brown, about 10 minutes.

TACOS IN A BAG

1 lb. Grass-fed Hamburger   Black Beans

Lettuce   Tomatoes

Tofutti Sour Cream   Salsa (GF)

1 package GF Taco Seasoning   Any Taco Toppings you like

Individual serving-size bags of organic corn chips

Mix the hamburger with one package of taco seasoning and cook according to package directions. Crush chips in bag. Cut the top off the chip bags and place meat, black beans, lettuce, tomatoes, salsa, and any other desired taco toppings in the bag, stir and eat. Use plastic spoons and there are no dishes to wash!

FRIED EGG SANDWICH

1 Egg   1 T. Coconut Oil

2 slices of GF Bread   GF Ketchup

Sea Salt and Pepper to taste

Melt coconut oil in a pan. Crack the egg, breaking the yolk, and cook over medium heat, flipping once, until completely done. Lightly smear ketchup on each slice of bread; place egg on sandwich, add sea salt and pepper, close and eat!

QUESADILLAS

Goat Gouda Cheese, grated   Chicken/Steak/Refried
  (Rice/Soy Cheddar)   or Black Beans (all optional)

Ivory Teff Tortillas or Brown   Guacamole (page 194)
  Rice Tortillas

Tofutti Sour Cream   GF Salsa

Spray a frying pan or griddle with olive oil. Place one tortilla in the pan and top with a thin layer of grated cheese, meat and/or beans, then a little more cheese. Top with another tortilla. Grill over medium heat until toasted golden brown and cheese is melting; flip and toast other side of tortilla. Remove from pan and slice with a pizza cutter into wedges. Serve with salsa, Tofutti sour cream, and guacamole for dipping.

◆Enrico's Salsa is a great brand you can find at most co-ops

BUILD-A-SUB

Sandwich Meat   GF Hot Dog Buns

GF Mayo, Mustard   GF Pickles

Lettuce   Tomato Slices

Onions, sliced in rings   Pepperoncini Peppers

Put all the sandwich toppings on the table and let your kids build their own sandwiches. They love to do this!

ORGANIC RED PEPPER TURKEY ROLLS

Deli Turkey slices GF   Organic Red Pepper strips
  (nitrite-free)   (thin)

◆Try Apple Gate Farms Deli Turkey slices

Wrap 1 slice of red pepper in a slice of turkey meat. For a fun option, I sometimes serve it with pizza sauce or spaghetti sauce for dipping.

PIZZA PACKS

GF Crackers – try Glutino   Pizza Sauce (page 163)

Slices of Goat Gouda or   Slices of NF Salami
  Cheddar Cheese   or Pepperoni

Take a cracker, put a spoonful of sauce on it, top with a slice of meat and cheese. Eat up!

Pizza Boats

Millet Hot Dog or GF Hot Dog
Bun of choice, cut in ½
the long way

Goat Gouda Cheese, grated
(Rice/Soy Mozzarella)

Pizza Sauce (page 163)

Favorite Pizza Toppings

Top each bun with sauce, desired toppings and cheese (my kids like to make their own). Bake in a 425-degree oven until cheese is melted and golden brown.

Incredible Tortilla Pizzas

Pepperoni GF (nitrite-free)

Pizza or Spaghetti Sauce
(pages 163 & 183)

Purple Onion slices

Sliced Garlic

Red and Green Pepper strips

Tomato Slices

Goat Garlic and Herb
Gouda Cheese slices
(Rice/Soy Mozzarella)

Brown Rice Tortillas

Place a tortilla on a cookie sheet or pizza stone. Cover with sauce, pepper slices, onion slices, garlic slices. Place in 375-degree oven; bake until veggies are tender, about 5-10 minutes. Put a layer of pepperoni (if desired), cheese, and top with tomato slices. Bake until melted and golden brown on top.

◆For a Tortilla Pizza use an ivory teff or brown rice tortilla as the crust.

PIZZA PARTY

Pepperoni GF (nitrite-free)
  Apple Gate Farms

Pizza or Spaghetti Sauce
  (pages 163 & 183)

Goat Gouda Cheese slices
  (Rice/Soy Mozzarella)

GF Crackers
  (Glutino's work best)

Stack a cracker with sauce, cheese, and a slice of pepperoni. Enjoy!

ENGLISH MUFFIN PIZZAS

1 Kinnikinnick Foods English
  Muffins

Grated Goat Gouda Cheese
  (Rice/Soy Mozzarella)

Grated Pecorino Cheese
  (Nutritional Yeast)

Pepperoni GF (nitrite-free)

Pizza or Spaghetti Sauce
  (pages 163 & 183)

Cut bagel in half. Top each half with a spoon of sauce, one slice pepperoni, and both cheeses. Bake in a 350-degree oven until cheese is golden brown.

PBJ or SBJ Tortillas

Take an ivory teff or brown rice tortilla and spread peanut or sun butter (any nut butter) on it. Next, spread fruit-sweetened jam/jelly over the top. Roll and eat! They are tasty with honey or agave instead of jam, as well – just a bit messier. This is great picnic food!

ITALIAN DIPPERS

Millet Hot Dog or GF Hot Dog
Bun, cut long way in half

Goat Gouda Cheese, grated
(Rice/Soy Mozzarella)

Spaghetti Sauce (page 183)

Top buns with cheese. Bake in 425-degree oven until cheese is melted and golden brown. Serve with a side of spaghetti sauce for dipping.

JEANNE'S PEANUT DIP OVER PASTA

⅔ c. Organic Creamy Peanut
Butter

¼ c. Honey or Maple Syrup

⅓ c. Brown Rice Vinegar

3 T. Water

2 T. Tamari GF Soy Sauce

1 T. fresh minced Ginger

2 cloves crushed Garlic

1½ tsp. toasted Sesame Oil

¼ tsp. crushed Red Pepper
Flakes (optional)

1 c. chopped Fresh Cilantro
(packed loosely)

1 box Rice Noodles

Cook brown rice noodles according to instructions on box. Combine all ingredients (except cilantro) in a blender and process until smooth. Add cilantro and pulse briefly until just chopped. Place noodles on plate and top with sauce. This dish can be served hot or cold.

✔ HEAD START TIP: *Keeps in fridge for 2-3 days in sealed container.*

BUILD YOUR OWN SALAD

Grape Tomatoes	Carrots, diced
Onions, diced	Cucumber slices
Peas	Hard Boiled Eggs
Goat Cheese Crumbles	Romaine or Leafy Green Lettuce

Place all the ingredients out and let your children top their salads with their favorite toppings. Top with favorite dressing. My children usually just use olive oil and balsamic vinegar. There are some dressing recipes in the back you can try. Drew's has a great Italian dressing that is DF/GF and you can find it at most co-ops.

MAC-N-CHEESE

1 package Brown Rice Noodles (cooked)	½ c. Grass-fed Butter or Earth Balance
½ c. Rice (or Almond) Milk	1 T. Cornstarch
½ to ¾ c. Pecorino Cheese (Soy or Rice Mozzarella)	Sea Salt to taste

Prepare noodles. As noodles cook, melt butter. Add in milk. Grate cheese. Add cheese and whisk until fully melted. Add cornstarch and whisk until thickened, 3-5 minutes. Pour cheese sauce over noodles. Season with sea salt to taste. Pepper adds a bit of spice if you would like a bit more of a kick.

Noodles & Cheese

½ c. (or more) Pecorino
  Cheese, grated or (Nutritional
  Yeast, just sprinkle on
  as desired)

Olive Oil

1 lb. Brown Rice Pasta
  Noodles

Cook noodles as directed on package. Strain noodles, place in large bowl and drizzle generously with olive oil. Sprinkle with cheese, stir, and serve.

Frittatas

Organic Corn Tortillas

1 (16 oz.) can GF Refried
  Beans

Olive Oil

GF Salsa

Tofutti Sour Cream

Diced Tomatoes

Diced Onion

Goat Gouda Cheese or Goat Cheddar, grated (Rice/Soy Cheddar)

Place about 1 T. of olive oil in a sauté pan. Heat slowly on medium heat, add 1 corn tortilla. Fry on one side until golden brown, flip and fry until other side is golden brown. Remove from heat. Top with heated refried beans, cheese, salsa, tomatoes, onion, and sour cream. (*You can add any other topping you would like as well: olives, black beans, cilantro, etc.*)

NOTES

DINNER RECIPES

Fresh Veggie Chili

3 cloves crushed Garlic

1 finely diced Organic Red Pepper

Sea Salt and Pepper to taste

2 tsp. Ground Cumin

2 quarts diced fresh or canned Tomatoes

1 finely diced Yellow Onion

1 finely diced Organic Green Pepper

2 T. Chili Powder (or more)

2 T. Olive Oil

1 c. GF Organic Chicken Broth

Place olive oil in a sauté pan. On medium heat, sauté garlic, onion, and peppers until tender, about 10 minutes. Add chili powder, cumin, salt and pepper, sauté one minute. Stir in tomatoes and chicken broth. Simmer for one hour or more to enhance flavor. For more zip, add more chili powder. For overall fuller flavor, add more sea salt.

Corn Bread

2 Organic Eggs

¼ c. Xylitol

1 c. Rice Milk

½ c. Millet Flour

⅔ c. Corn Meal

¼ tsp. Baking Soda

¾ tsp. Sea Salt

1 T. Honey

½ c. Brown Rice Flour

2 tsp. Baking Powder

¼ c. Earth Balance Stick

Preheat oven to 400 degrees. Butter an 8 x 8 x 2 inch baking dish. Beat eggs in large bowl. Add xylitol and honey. In a small bowl mix flours, corn meal, baking powder, baking soda, and sea salt. Add dry ingredients and milk, alternating, into the egg mixture. When well mixed, add melted Earth Balance and pour into baking dish. Bake 20-30 minutes or until toothpick comes out clean.

CORN BREAD W/MAPLE BUTTER SPREAD

1 c. Corn Meal	½ c. Millet
½ c. Brown Rice Flour	2 Organic Eggs
¼ c. Olive Oil	2 tsp. Baking Powder
½ tsp. Baking Soda	¼ c. Honey
¾ tsp. Sea Salt	1 c. Rice Milk w/1 T. Lemon Juice in it

Spray 1 loaf pan (or 12 muffin cups) with an olive oil spray. Preheat oven to 425 degrees. In a large bowl combine corn meal, flour, baking powder, salt and baking soda. In a small bowl, whisk together rice milk, eggs, honey, and oil. When well mixed, stir into dry ingredients. Pour into pan or muffin tins and bake until golden brown, about 15 minutes.

MAPLE BUTTER SPREAD: With an electric mixer, whip 1/2 c. whipped Earth Balance or grass-fed butter with 1/4 c. pure maple syrup.

CHILI #1

1 lb. Ground Beef, Buffalo, or Venison

1 (15.5 oz.) can Dark Red Kidney Beans or Black Beans

1 (32 oz.) can diced Tomatoes

1 large Onion, diced fine

GF Organic Ketchup (to taste)

1 T. Chili Powder

Sauté meat and diced onions in a large stockpot. When done, add beans with juice and tomatoes with juice. Add ketchup and chili powder to taste. Simmer 1 hour.

✔ HEAD START TIP: *The chili recipes work to put in a crock-pot and cook all day (8 or more hours) on low for an easy dinner – all ready to go! They also freeze well for quick weeknight meals.*

CHILI #2

1 lb. Ground Beef or Buffalo

1 large Onion

2 cloves crushed Garlic

3 T. Organic GF Ketchup

2 (15oz) cans Organic Black Beans

1 T. Chili Powder

1 T. Ground Cumin

2 tsp. Sea Salt

2 (32oz) cans Diced Tomatoes

✱ TRICKY MOM'S TIP: *Put any or all of the following ingredients into a food processor and puree into a paste consistency: zucchini, carrots, peppers, celery, broccoli, or cauliflower, and secretly add it to your chili.*

In large stockpot, sauté beef/buffalo, diced onion, and garlic. When meat is fully cooked, add beans with juice, tomatoes with juice, ketchup, chili powder, cumin and sea salt. Simmer 1 or more hours. Serve over cooked brown rice. Top with cheese of choice (goat cheddar/Gouda, rice or soy-cheddar) and Tofutti sour cream.

Burrito Bowls

COOKED BROWN RICE: Enough for 1 serving per person. Prepare according to directions on package.

FILLINGS OF CHOICE:

Diced peppers, cooked taco/fajita meat, beans, rice, salsa, guacamole, onions, green pepper, goat Gouda or cheddar (rice or soy cheddar) cheese, lettuce, tomatoes, Tofutti sour cream, cilantro, salsa, etc.

Place a layer of brown rice in the bottom of a bowl. Place your favorite toppings on the rice. Enjoy!

Stir Fry

4 boneless skinless Chicken Breasts, cooked and cubed	2-3 T. GF Tamari Soy Sauce or GF Teriyaki Sauce
2 bags Frozen Vegetables	1 tsp. Sesame Oil
2 T. Olive Oil	Cooked Brown Jasmine Rice (per directions on package)

Heat olive oil and sesame oil in deep fry pan on medium heat. Add both bags of vegetables and stir-fry until tender. Add cooked chicken. Add 2-3 T. of soy sauce or teriyaki sauce, and stir to mix. Cook until heated through. Add more soy or teriyaki sauce to taste if desired. Serve over rice.

QUINOA & BLACK BEANS

¾ cup Quinoa

1 chopped Onion

1½ c. GF Chicken Broth

1 tsp. Ground Cumin

Sea Salt & Pepper

2 (15oz.) cans Black Beans
  (drained and rinsed)

1 tsp. Olive Oil

3 cloves crushed Garlic

1 c. frozen Organic Corn

¼ tsp. Cayenne Pepper

½ c. chopped fresh Cilantro

Soak quinoa for 5 minutes in cold water and drain. Heat oil in sauce-pan on low. Sauté onion and garlic until tender. Add quinoa, broth, cumin, cayenne, salt and pepper. Bring to a boil, reduce heat and simmer, covered, for 20 minutes. Add frozen corn and cilantro. Serve over brown rice, topped with Tofutti sour cream and salsa.

TOMATO BASIL WILD-CAUGHT SALMON

1 c. fresh Basil

2 T. crushed Garlic

1 Fillet Wild-Caught Salmon

⅔ c. GF Organic Chicken Broth

½ c. Sun Dried Tomatoes

¼ c. Olive Oil

2 T. Organic Lemon Juice

Place the basil, tomatoes, garlic, and olive oil into a blender and puree until smooth. In a large sauté pan, combine the chicken broth and lemon juice, allow to simmer on low while you cut salmon into desired serving sizes, coat with puree on both sides of fish and place in pan. Braise (spoon chicken broth/lemon juice mixture over the fish) until tender and flakes with a fork. DO NOT FLIP THE FISH.

GRILLED OR BROILED WILD-CAUGHT SALMON

2 Lemons   Garlic Salt, Pepper

1 Whole Wild-Caught Salmon Filet

To GRILL: Prepare grill to medium high heat. Cover the grate with a piece of aluminum foil. Cut a piece of parchment paper a little larger than your salmon fillet and place on the foil, then place fillet on parchment paper. Season each side of salmon with fresh squeezed lemon juice (1 lemon per side), and garlic salt and pepper to taste. Grill for about 10-15 minutes, flip and continue to grill until fish flakes easily with a fork.

To BROIL: Move oven rack to top position. Preheat oven to low broil. Season fish with lemon juice (1 lemon per side), garlic salt and pepper to taste. Put under broiler for about 10-15 minutes, flip and continue to broil until fish flakes easily with a fork.

BBQ RIBS

¾ c. GF Ketchup   ½ c. Pure Maple Syrup

3 T. Apple Cider Vinegar   1 Rack of Ribs
     (Any bone-in variety will work, or country boneless style)

Place 1 inch of water in the bottom of a roasting pan and add ribs. Place in a 350-degree oven for one hour. Remove from oven and baste both sides of ribs with BBQ sauce.

To GRILL: Place on broiling pan and broil on low until browned, about 5 minutes per side.

To BROIL: Grill over medium heat until browned, about 5 minutes per side.

Pizza Sauce

28 oz. can Diced Tomatoes (or fresh)

3 cloves crushed Garlic

½ tsp. Sea Salt

¼ tsp. Pepper

1 ½ tsp. Dried Basil

1 tsp. Dried Oregano

½ tsp. Fennel

Olive Oil

◆If your kids don't like chunky sauce, put in blender and puree.

Pour a layer of olive oil in a large saucepan, heat to medium heat and add garlic; sauté until golden brown. Add tomatoes with juices and seasonings. Cook for 15 minutes.

✔ HEAD START TIP: *The sauce freezes well.*

HOME MADE PIZZA

Pizza Crust Mix or Frozen Pre-Made GF Crust

GF Pepperoni (nitrite-free)

1 c. or more Goat Gouda (Rice or Soy Mozzarella)

½ c. grated Pecorino or (a sprinkling of Nutritional Yeast)

(Pizza sauce recipe above.) Smear some sauce on the crust, add pepperoni, and top with cheese – and any other pizza toppings your family enjoys. Bake at 425 degrees until cheese is golden brown and bubbly.

CHINESE BEEF ROAST

3 lb. Beef Roast   Sea Salt & Pepper
  (Arm or Rump)

1 tsp. Ground Ginger   2 large sliced Red Onions

½ c. GF Soy Sauce   ½ c. Water

Pour water into pot. Season entire roast liberally with sea salt and pepper, and place in crock-pot. Pour soy sauce over roast and sprinkle with ginger. Spread onions all over roast. Cover and cook on low for 8-10 hours.

BEEF, TOMATOES & NOODLE HOT DISH

1½ lb. Stew Meat   ¼ c. Millet Flour

2 c. diced Tomatoes   1 tsp. Sea Salt

½ tsp. Pepper   1 medium Onion, diced

1 lb. cooked Brown Rice Noodles

Toss stew meat in flour and place in crock-pot. Add tomatoes, salt, pepper, and onion, and enough water to cover. Cook on low for 6-8 hours and serve over cooked pasta.

ROAST BEEF w/VEGGIES

3-4 lb. Roast (of any kind)   4 Organic Potatoes

6 Carrots   2 Ribs Celery

2 large Purple Onions

Season a roast on both sides with garlic salt and pepper. Pour 1-2 inches of water in bottom of roaster and place roast in roasting pan. Cut up the following veggies in one-inch chunks and place around roast: potatoes, carrots, celery, and onion. Bake at 350 degrees for about 1½ to 2 hours until done according to meat thermometer – see page for desired doneness temperature.

CHERYL'S DONE-AT-NOON BEEF STEW

5 Carrots, chopped   1 Rutabaga (optional)
 (1 inch pieces)   Chopped (1 inch pieces)

2 Onions, chopped   1 can Water

3 chopped Parsnips   3 stalks Celery, chopped
 (1 inch pieces)   (1 inch)

2 cans crushed Tomatoes   1 lb. cubed Stew Beef

Place raw cubed meat into Dutch oven or roaster. Toss in all the chopped veggies. Pour in the water, stir in tomatoes and cover. Place in oven at 275 degrees at noon and bake until dinnertime. Do not open lid until ready to eat.

HAMBURGER HOT DISH

1 lb. Grass-fed Ground Beef

Sea Salt & Pepper

2 (32 oz) cans of diced Tomatoes OR fresh

16 oz box of Rice Elbow Noodles

1 diced Medium Yellow Onion

Pecorino Cheese – Optional (Nutritional Yeast)

Brown the ground beef and onion in a large frying pan. Drain off fat. As beef is cooking, prepare one box of elbow noodles according to box directions. In a large casserole dish, mix beef, cooked noodles, diced tomatoes, and season with salt and pepper to taste. Place in a 350-degree oven and bake for 45 minutes until heated through. Serve topped with grated pecorino cheese or Nutritional Yeast if desired.

GRILLED SIRLOIN STEAK W/GARLIC BUTTER

Grass-fed Beef Top Sirloin Steaks

½ c. Earth Balance or Grass-fed Butter

2 tsp. Garlic Powder

Sea Salt & Pepper to taste

4 cloves minced Garlic

Put gas grill on high or prepare charcoal grill for direct cooking. In small saucepan, melt Earth Balance over medium heat. Add garlic powder and minced garlic, whisk with fork. Set aside. Sprinkle both sides of steak with salt and pepper. Grill steaks 4-5 minutes per side or to desired doneness. Allow to rest for 3 minutes and then serve steak brushed liberally with garlic sauce.

STIR-FRIED STEAK & RICE

Brown Rice	1 1b. Flank Steak
2 cloves crushed Garlic	¼ c. GF Tamari Soy Sauce
2 tsp. Cornstarch	1 tsp. Raw Sugar
2 tsp. Sesame Oil	3 T. Coconut Oil
3 T. chopped Peanuts	¼ c. fresh Cilantro
2 c. fresh Sugar Snap Peas, trimmed (or 8 oz. Frozen Pea Pods – thawed)	½ tsp. crushed Red Pepper (Optional)

Cook rice according to directions (one serving per person). Cut steak across the grain into 1-inch thick slices. Combine steak, garlic, and pepper in a bowl and toss to coat. In a separate bowl combine soy sauce, cornstarch, and sugar; whisk until smooth. Heat coconut oil in pan over medium high heat. Add snap peas and stir-fry about 1 minute until heated through. Add meat mixture to pan and stir-fry until meat is cooked through, about 2 minutes. Add soy sauce mixture to pan and stir-fry for about 1 minute or until sauce thickens. Serve over rice. Top with chopped cilantro and chopped peanuts.

SPICY FRENCH DIP SANDWICHES

3-4 lb Beef Roast	GF Hot Dog Buns
1 large jar Pepperoncini Peppers	

Place roast in crock-pot. Pour entire jar of pepperoncini peppers with juice on the roast. Cook on low for up to 12 hours (you can dilute the potency with water, if you like it a bit less spicy). Serve on toasted individual sized hot dog buns. Use the juice at the bottom of the crock-pot as an au jus for dipping.

Grandma Anita's Brisket

1 medium sized Brisket	½ tsp. celery salt
½ tsp. garlic salt	½ tsp. onion powder
¼ c. GF Liquid Smoke	

Lay a large piece of aluminum foil on your work surface. Place a same-size piece of parchment paper on top of it. Put brisket in the center of the parchment paper. Sprinkle with GF liquid smoke, celery & garlic salt, onion powder. Wrap with parchment so all meat is covered and then wrap foil around to seal. Place in crock-pot on low for 8-12 hours.

French Dip Sandwiches

3-4 lb. Beef Roast	1 tsp. Sea Salt
1 tsp. White Pepper	1 T. Dried Rosemary
1 T. Dried Oregano	1 T. Garlic Powder
1 c. Water	GF Hot Dog Buns

Place water and beef in crock-pot. Sprinkle with salt, white pepper, rosemary, oregano, and garlic powder. Cook on low for 6-7 hours. Remove the meat and shred. Serve on toasted individual sized hot dog buns. Use the juice at the bottom of the crock-pot as an au jus for dipping.

GRILLED FLANK STEAK

¼ c. Organic Orange Juice

2 T. fresh Lime Juice

¾ tsp. Sea Salt

1½ lb. Flank Steak

1 tsp. minced Garlic

1 tsp. Ground Cumin

½ tsp. Pepper

Combine orange juice, lime juice, and garlic in a small bowl. Add cumin, salt, and pepper to the juice mixture. Place steak in a large resealable bag and pour juice mixture over the meat. Seal the bag and marinate in the fridge for about 20 minutes. Preheat broiler or grill. Broil or grill each side of steak for about 6 minutes per side or to desired doneness.

LITTLE CHEDDAR MEAT LOAVES

MEAT:

1 lb. Grass-fed Ground Beef

1 Organic Egg

¾ c. Rice Milk

1 c. Goat Cheddar Cheese
(Rice or Soy)

½ c. GF Oats

½ c. finely diced Onion

1 tsp. Sea Salt

SAUCE:

⅔ c. GF Ketchup

¼ c. Organic Brown Sugar
or Maple Syrup

1½ tsp. GF Mustard

Preheat oven to 350 degrees. In a large bowl, mix ground beef, egg, milk, cheese, sea salt, oats, and onion. Divide into 8 equal portions, shape into 8 individual loaves, and place in 9 x 13 pan. Mix sauce ingredients and spoon over each loaf. Place in oven and bake for about 45 minutes.

CROCK-POT DILLED ROAST

1 tsp. Sea Salt	¼ tsp. Pepper
2 tsp. Dill Weed	¼ c. Water
1 T. Apple Cider Vinegar	½ c. Water
1 c. Tofutti Sour Cream	½ Onion, sliced
3 T. Corn Starch or Arrowroot 3-4 lb. Beef Roast (Arm/Rump)	2 cloves Garlic

Sprinkle both sides of roast with salt, pepper, and dill weed. Place in crock-pot. Add ¼ c. water, vinegar, and onion. Cook 7-9 hours. Remove meat from crock-pot and turn crock-pot to high (cover meat to keep warm). Dissolve cornstarch in ½ c. water. Stir cornstarch mixture into meat drippings in crock-pot, cook on high for 5 minutes, stir in sour cream, cook on high another 5 minutes.

◆ If gravy does not thicken, remove it from your crock-pot and put it in a skillet and heat – it will then thicken. Sometimes the crock-pot doesn't get it hot enough to thicken.

CURRIED CHICKEN

4 Chicken Breasts	Zest & Juice of 1 Organic Orange
3 T. Olive Oil	1 cup Coconut Milk
1 Onion, diced	1 cup Organic Chicken Broth
2 cloves crushed Garlic	2 T. Mango Chutney
1 T. Curry Powder	1 T. chopped Cilantro
1 T. fresh grated Ginger	1 cup Frozen Peas or Broccoli Florets
¼ c. toasted slivered Almonds	Sea Salt & Pepper

Put chicken in deep sauté pan and cover with water. Boil until cooked through. Remove from water and dice into bite-size pieces. Remove water from pan, wash and dry. Place olive oil in pan and heat slowly. Sauté onion until tender. Add garlic, sauté briefly. Add curry, ginger, orange zest, and juice and stir. Stir in coconut milk and broth; bring to a boil. Reduce heat to low, add chicken, peas and/or broccoli and cook until chicken is heated through, about 5 minutes. Stir in chutney. Serve over brown rice. Sprinkle cilantro and almonds on top.

TERIYAKI MEAT MARINADE

¼ c. GF Soy Sauce	1 clove pressed Garlic
3 T. Honey	1½ tsp. Ground Ginger
2 T. Apple Cider Vinegar	¾ c. Olive Oil

This is good for beef or chicken. In a small bowl, mix ingredients. Put meat into a large resealable bag, pour marinade over meat and close bag. Place in refrigerator for about 24 hours, turn occasionally. Place marinated meat on broiling pan and broil on high until done. (Beef is done when it reaches 155 degrees, chicken at 170 degrees.)

SERVING SUGGESTIONS:

Place marinated meat on grill and grill until done.

OR: Skewer as a kabob with veggies and grill.

OR: Cut meat in bite-size pieces and sauté with veggies. Serve over brown rice.

CROCK-POT CHICKEN & POTATOES

4-6 Potatoes – cut in quarters	1 Whole Chicken
2 Large Onions - Yellow	1 T. crushed Garlic
3 tsp. Dried Oregano	1 tsp. Sea Salt
½ tsp. Pepper	1 T. Olive Oil

Place potatoes in bottom of crock-pot, place chicken on top of potatoes drizzle with olive oil, place onions on top of chicken, sprinkle all of it with oregano, salt, garlic, and pepper. Cover and cook on high for 5-6 hours or low for 9-10 hours.

THAI CHICKEN SATAY

1½ lbs. Chicken Tenders	½ c. Arrowroot Powder
2 T. Fish Sauce	2 T. Coconut Oil
1 large Onion	2 tsp. minced Garlic
1 tsp. Ground Ginger	½ c. Coconut Milk
1 T. Xylitol	1 T. Organic Lime Juice
Brown Rice	

Prepare desired amount of brown rice according to the directions on the package. Put fish sauce in a small bowl. Spread arrowroot powder on a plate. Dip each chicken tender in fish sauce and then coat in arrowroot. Place in sauté pan that has 2 T. of heated coconut oil in it (add more oil as needed for frying). Sauté on medium high heat for 5 minutes. Remove from pan. Heat another 1 T. coconut oil in skillet. Add sliced onion, garlic, and ground ginger, sauté for 1 minute. Stir in chicken and cook until done. Stir in coconut milk, xylitol, and lime juice. Cook until heated through. Serve over rice and top each serving with cilantro.

SWEET & SPICY CHICKEN STRIPS

4 boneless, skinless chicken breasts

2 T. Honey

¼ c. GF Tamari Soy Sauce

2 tsp. chopped Garlic

2 T. chopped fresh Ginger Root

1 T. Olive Oil

1 T. Maple Syrup

Sea Salt & Pepper

Slice chicken into strips. Mix syrup, honey, soy sauce, ginger, and garlic together. Lightly salt and pepper chicken strips. Heat oil on medium heat in large skillet. Brown chicken strips about 1 minute on each side. Pour sauce over chicken and cook 8-10 minutes until sauce cooks down and coats chicken strips. This can be served as a main course meat, but I like to serve it over rice and veggies like an Asian bowl. I sauté up some Asian veggies and then layer rice, veggies, and top with meat!

SWEET & SOUR CHICKEN

4 Chicken Breasts (hormone and antibiotic free)

BREADING:

2 Organic Eggs

½ c. Cornstarch

¼ tsp. Garlic Salt

Sauce:

¾ c. Raw Sugar (Turbinado)

½ c. Apple Cider Vinegar

4 T. GF Ketchup

1 T. GF Soy Sauce

Preheat oven to 350 degrees. Dice chicken into 1-inch pieces. Beat eggs in a bowl. Place cornstarch on a large plate and sprinkle garlic salt over cornstarch, toss with fork to blend. Dip chicken pieces into egg and then roll in cornstarch. Heat oil in a large saucepan on medium high heat. Place breaded chicken directly into frying pan. When golden brown on all sides, place in large baking dish with cover. In a small saucepan over medium heat, cook sugar, vinegar, ketchup, and soy sauce, stirring until sugar dissolves. Pour over chicken in baking dish. Cover and bake for about 1 hour.

ROASTED CHICKEN W/VEGGIES

1 Whole Chicken	4 Organic Potatoes
6 Carrots	2 ribs of Celery
1 large Purple Onion	Garlic Salt
1 small to medium Yellow Onion	Pepper

Peel one small to medium onion. Clean and rinse chicken. Place onion in cavity of chicken. Liberally season outside of chicken with garlic salt and pepper. Rub olive oil over entire chicken. Pour 1-2 inches of water in bottom of roasting pan. Place prepared chicken into roasting pan. Cut up the following veggies in one-inch chunks and place around the chicken: potatoes, carrots, celery, and onion. Cover and place in a 350-degree oven. Bake for about one hour, remove cover and bake another 30-60 minutes until golden brown (baste as needed) and done according to meat thermometer.

SESAME CHICKEN STRIPS

½ c. Honey   ¼ c. GF Tamari Soy Sauce

1 T. Lemon Juice   ½ c. Sesame Seeds

2 lbs. boneless, skinless
  Chicken Breast, cut in strips

Place chicken strips in a 9 x 13 pan. In a bowl mix honey, soy sauce, lemon juice, and sesame seeds. Pour over chicken and stir to coat well. Bake at 350 degrees for about 45 minutes or until chicken is fully cooked and coated with sauce.

JEANNE'S PEANUT DIP w/CHICKEN OVER PASTA

¼ c. Honey or Maple Syrup   ⅓ c. Brown Rice Vinegar

3 T. Water   2 T. GF Soy Sauce

1 T. fresh minced Ginger   2 cloves crushed Garlic

1½ tsp. toasted Sesame Oil   1 box Rice Noodles

¼ tsp. crushed Red Pepper   1 c. chopped fresh Cilantro
  Flakes – optional   (packed loosely)

Cooked & Diced Chicken   ⅔ c. Organic Creamy
  Breast   Peanut Butter

Cook noodles according to instructions on box. Combine all ingredients (except cilantro and chicken) in a blender and process until smooth. Add cilantro and pulse briefly until just chopped. Place the noodles on plate, top with chicken and sauce. This dish can be served hot or cold.

OVEN ROASTED DIJON CHICKEN

4 boneless Chicken Breasts (hormone/antibiotic-free)

MARINADE:

5 tsp. GF Dijon Mustard	1 clove fresh crushed Garlic
1 stick – Earth Balance or Grass-fed Butter	

BREADING:

1½ cup GF Corn Flake Crumbs	5 T. shredded Pecorino Cheese (Nutritional Yeast)
2 T. fresh or dried Parsley, Minced	

FOR MARINADE: Melt Earth Balance or butter in sauté pan over low heat. Add garlic and simmer on low heat for five minutes, being careful not to let it burn. Blend in mustard and stir well. Remove from heat and let cool, but not enough to solidify. When cool, whip vigorously until mixture thickens.

FOR BREADING: Mix together all ingredients, blending well, and pour onto a large plate.

Preheat oven to 350 degrees. Dip chicken breasts into Earth Balance mixture, then in breading mixture, packing crumbs onto chicken to coat well. Place prepared chicken breasts on a sheet pan (cookie sheet). Place in oven and bake for about 40 minutes until meat thermometer reads 170 degrees.

BAKED SPAGHETTI

◆ *This can't be done 100% dairy-free*

1 lb. GF Spaghetti Noodles

4 oz. crumbled Goat Cheese

1 c. grated Organic Mozzarella
(or Goat Gouda)

1 jar Spaghetti Sauce

1 Organic Egg

½ c. grated Pecorino Cheese

Prepare noodles according to package directions. Strain noodles and place in a large bowl. In a small bowl mix together ricotta and egg. Add mozzarella and pecorino and stir well. Pour cheese mixture into noodles and mix with hands until all noodles are coated. Grease two loaf pans and equally divide noodle mixture into each pan. Press down in pan and bake in a 350-degree oven for about 30 minutes or until it begins to brown on top. Allow to cool a few minutes before slicing like bread. Serve with warmed spaghetti sauce ladled over the top.

BAKED ZITI

◆ *This can't be done 100% dairy-free*

2 jars Spaghetti Sauce
(or homemade)

4 oz. crumbled Goat Cheese

½ c. grated Pecorino Cheese

1 c. grated Tomato Basil
Goat Cheese

1 lb. Rice Penne Noodles

Prepare noodles according to package directions. Pour spaghetti sauce, goat crumbles, Gouda, and pecorino into a 9 x 13 pan and mix thoroughly. Stir in cooked noodles and place in preheated 350-degree oven. Bake about 30 minutes until heated through.

LINGUINE w/ROASTED RED PEPPERS, PEAS & PINE NUTS

From *Simple Vegetarian Pleasures* by Jeanne Lemlin

1 lb. GF Spaghetti or Linguine Noodles	¾ c. roasted Red Peppers, diced
⅓ c. Olive Oil	4 cloves Garlic, crushed
2 T. Pine Nuts	1½ c. Peas
½ tsp. Sea Salt (or to taste)	Pepper to taste
½ c. fresh Parsley (or 1 tsp. dried)	⅓ c. grated Pecorino Cheese

Cook noodles according to package. While noodles cook, heat olive oil in a skillet. Add garlic and toast. When brown, stir in peppers, pine nuts, peas, salt, pepper and cook 1 minute, stirring often. Remove ¼ cup of starch water from noodles and add it to the sauce along with the parsley. Drain noodles. Place in large bowl, pour sauce over noodles and toss, top with cheese. Serve!

ASIAN CHICKEN WINGS "DRUMMIES"

Family Pack of Chicken Drummies or Wings	1¼ c. Water
15 T. GF Tamari Soy Sauce	1 clove crushed Garlic
1 Green Onion, chopped	¼ c. Sesame Oil

Mix water, garlic, soy sauce, onion and sesame oil in a 9 x 13 pan. Add chicken. Bake at 350 degrees until sauce cooks down and coats chicken – about 1 hour.

DAIRY-FREE STUFFED JUMBO SHELLS

◆*For 100% dairy-free: Use 3 c. Rice or Soy Mozzarella and 1 T. of Nutritional Yeast in place of other cheese. Add egg. Mix well and stuff shells.*

1 (8oz.) package of GF Jumbo Shells	1 lb. GF Italian Sausage (optional)
½ c. chopped Onion	2 cloves crushed Garlic
1 (28 oz.) can diced Tomatoes	1 (6oz.) can Tomato Paste
1 tsp. dried Basil	½ tsp. Sea Salt
¼ tsp. Pepper	1 Organic Egg
(4 oz.) Goat Feta or Goat Crumbles	1 c. grated Tomato Basil Goat Cheese
2 c. grated Goat Gouda	⅓ c. grated Pecorino Romano (Sheep)

Cook noodles according to directions on package. Preheat oven to 350 degrees.

SAUCE: In a large skillet brown sausage (if using) and pour off fat. If not using meat, just sauté veggies in olive oil. Add onion and garlic and cook until tender. Stir in tomatoes, tomato paste, basil, salt, and pepper. Bring to a boil and then reduce heat and simmer for at least 15 minutes, uncovered.

Filling: In a medium bowl combine 1 c. goat Gouda, all other cheeses and egg and mix well. Stuff cheese mixture into each cooked noodle.

Spread half the sauce on the bottom of a 9 x 13 pan. Place stuffed noodles on top of sauce. Spoon remaining sauce over noodles. Cover and bake 35 minutes or until hot and bubbly. Uncover and top with remaining 1 c. goat Gouda cheese. Bake 5 minutes longer.

JEANNE'S RATATOUILLE

◆ *To maximize flavor, dice all veggies <u>very fine</u>!*

1 medium Eggplant	Sea Salt & Black Pepper
¼ c. Olive Oil	2 cloves crushed Garlic
2 medium Purple Onions	3 small Zucchini
3 small Yellow Zucchini	2 Red Peppers
2 Yellow Peppers	¼ c. finely chopped Basil
Grated Pecorino Romano Cheese or (Nutritional Yeast) – optional	1 (28oz.) can Italian Plum Tomatoes

✔ HEAD START TIP: *This makes a LOT – freeze the leftovers for quick weeknight meals.*

In large stockpot, heat oil and garlic over medium heat. Add onion, zucchini, peppers, and eggplant. Cook, stirring occasionally, until all veggies are softened, about 10 minutes. Add tomatoes with juices. Add salt and pepper to taste. Simmer uncovered until all veggies are tender, about 30 minutes or longer. Stir in basil and adjust salt and pepper to taste. Serve immediately or at room temperature. Top with pecorino cheese or a sprinkle of Nutritional Yeast if desired. It's also delicious topped with a fried egg. To store, let cool and refrigerate in a sealed container – freezes well.

HIDDEN VEGGIE LASAGNA

1 box GF Lasagna Noodles

¾ c. diced Purple Onion

1 c. grated Tomato Basil
Goat Cheese

2 Red or Yellow Peppers

2 c. diced Eggplant

⅓ c. grated Pecorino Cheese

¼ tsp. Pepper

8 oz. Goat Crumbles

2 tsp. crushed Garlic

⅓ c. Rice Milk

½ tsp. chopped Oregano
Leaves

½ tsp. Sea Salt

2 jars Spaghetti Sauce

1 T. Olive Oil

2 c. chopped Zucchini

1 Organic Egg

Sauté garlic, onion, oregano, peppers, sea salt, pepper, in olive oil until tender. Add eggplant and zucchini for about 10 minutes. In a bowl whisk goat crumbles, egg, and rice milk until smooth. Layer the following in a 9 x 13 pan: ⅓ noodles, ⅓ sauce, ⅓ veggies, ⅓ cheese rice milk mixture, ⅓ grated tomato basil goat cheese, ⅓ grated pecorino cheese. Bake at 350 degrees for about 30-45 minutes.

TOMATO BASIL TART

1 Bob's Red Mill Biscuit Mix
(follow recipe for pie crust
on package)

5 Plum Tomatoes

½ c. Spectrum Canola Mayo
or Vegenaise

4 cloves crushed Garlic

1 brick grated Goat Gouda/
Mozzarella/Tomato Basil
(Rice or Soy – Mozzarella)

1 c. chopped Basil

¼ c. grated Pecorino Cheese
(1 tsp. Nutritional Yeast)

Prepare crust according to directions on package and place in pie pan. Poke bottom of crust with a fork multiple times – bake 10 minutes in 350-degree oven. Remove from oven (raise temperature of oven to 375 degrees) and sprinkle ½ of goat cheese (rice/soy) on bottom of crust. Cut tomatoes in ¼ inch slices and arrange evenly over the cheese. In a bowl mix the remaining Gouda (rice/soy), basil, mayo, pecorino (NY), and garlic. Spread this mixture over tomatoes. Bake at 375 degrees for about 30 minutes until heated through and golden brown.

HOMEMADE LOADED SPAGHETTI SAUCE

✔ HEAD START TIP: *This is great for freezing.*

⅓ c. Olive Oil	1 tsp. Sea Salt
2 Onions, diced	2 grated Carrots
½ tsp. Pepper	10 cloves crushed Garlic
1 tsp. Dried Oregano	1 Red Pepper
2 T. fresh diced Italian Parsley	Handful chopped fresh Basil
1 Zucchini (chopped)	1 quart diced Tomatoes
3 (15oz.) cans Tomato Sauce	

Chop all veggies into ½-inch chunks and sauté in olive oil at moderate heat until soft, about 25 minutes. Let cool. Stir in one quart of diced tomatoes. Ladle 1 scoop of tomato/veggie mixture into blender and puree until smooth, pour into stockpot. Repeat until all veggies are pureed. Add tomato sauce to pot. Add spices and let simmer on low for at least 1 hour. Serve over any kind of pasta or use it in any Italian dishes calling for a red sauce.

Enchiladas

1 T. Earth Balance or Grass-fed Butter

¾ c. Brown Rice Flour

3 T. chili powder

1 block Goat Gouda Cheese, shredded (or Rice/Soy Cheddar)

Ivory Teff or Brown Rice Tortillas

5 c. GF Organic Chicken Broth

1 (8oz.) can Tomato Sauce

1 (15 oz.) can Black Beans

Chicken/Beef – *optional*

1 c. cooked Brown Rice

Step 1: Sauce

Melt Earth Balance in a large saucepan. In a separate bowl mix flour and chili powder, whisk into melted Earth Balance. Whisk in tomato sauce. Pour in chicken broth and stir. Simmer for about 20 minutes, stirring occasionally to desired thickness. (Make multiple batches and freeze for the future – freezes well!)

Step 2: Tortilla Rolls

Prepare meat if using, mix meat, rice, beans together. Place 2 T. or so of rice mixture on edge of tortilla, and roll tight. Place seam down in a 9 x 13 pan that has been sprayed with olive oil. Pour sauce over tortillas, top with cheese and bake until bubbling in a 350-degree oven, about 30-45 minutes.

SPINACH & ROASTED RED PEPPER ENCHILADAS

FILLING:

8 oz. crumbled Goat Cheese

10 oz. box of frozen chopped Spinach, thawed

1 T. Olive Oil

1 tsp. Ground Cumin

½ tsp. Sea Salt

1 tsp. Dried Oregano

3 T. Rice Milk

7 oz. jar Roasted Red Peppers

1 medium Onion, diced

2 T. Pecorino Cheese (patted dry and diced)

Pepper to taste

8 GF Tortillas

THE SAUCE:

1¼ c. GF Salsa

¼ c. Rice Milk

½ c. Tofutti Sour Cream

TOPPING:

1¼ c. grated Goat Gouda Cheese

Puree goat cheese and rice milk in a blender until smooth. Place spinach in strainer and press out extra water, set aside. Heat olive oil on medium heat in a skillet, add onion and cook until soft, about 10 minutes. Add cumin and cook about 2 minutes to toast it. Stir in spinach, cook 2 minutes. Let mixture cool, then stir in goat cheese mixture and all other filling ingredients. Preheat oven to 385 degrees. Grease 9 x 13 pan. Divide spinach mixture onto the 8 tortillas, roll, and place in greased pan, seam down, packing them tightly in the dish. Make sauce by combining salsa, rice milk, and sour cream. Pour over enchiladas and top with cheese. Place in oven and bake for about 25 minutes until cheese is lightly brown and bubbly, heated through! Let set for 5 minutes before cutting and serving.

Vegetable Fried Rice

¼ cup finely diced Onion   3 Organic Eggs (beaten)

2½ cups cooked Brown Rice   Sea Salt & Pepper

1½ T. GF Soy Sauce   1-2 T. Olive Oil

1 c. Peas & Carrots or any frozen Veggie Mix

In a large frying pan pour olive oil and put to medium heat; sauté onions until tender, about 3 minutes. Add eggs and stir constantly, like scrambled eggs. Stir in rice, soy sauce, and salt and pepper to taste. Add veggies, cover loosely, and cook for 10 minutes, stir often to prevent burning.

Buffalo Chicken Wings "Drummies"

Family Pack of Chicken   GF Hot Sauce
Drummies or Wings

Take a 9 x 13 pan and place chicken in it. Pour hot sauce over top. Cook in 350-degree oven until chicken is done. If you want it hotter, marinate the chicken in hot sauce for a few hours or overnight.

NOTES

SOUPS

ASPARAGUS SOUP

8 T. Earth Balance or Grass-fed Butter

8 c. GF Organic Chicken Broth

2 lb. Asparagus

4 c. Yellow Onion, diced

½ c. Rice Milk or Almond Milk

Pecorino Cheese (Nutritional Yeast) – *optional*

Sea Salt & Pepper

✔ HEAD START TIP: *This freezes very well for quick lunches and dinners*

Melt Earth Balance in a stockpot, add onions and cook until tender. Add chicken broth. Clean asparagus, and cut in one-inch pieces. Place all but the tips in the pot. Cook 15-20 minutes until asparagus is tender. Puree in batches in blender and return to pot. Add tips and cook 10 minutes. Stir in rice milk. Season with salt and pepper to taste. Serve topped with pecorino cheese (Nutritional Yeast) – optional.

HAMBURGER SOUP

2 (32 oz.) cans crushed Tomatoes or fresh

1 lb. Grass-fed Hamburger

1 large Onion diced

3 large Carrots chopped

3 stalks Celery chopped

3 Organic Potatoes chopped

Brown beef with onion until fully cooked in a stock/soup pan. Add tomatoes, carrots, celery, and potatoes. Simmer until veggies are tender, about 1 hour. To speed up cooking, raise temperature.

Eggplant Tomato Soup

✱ Tricky Mom's Tip: *Make sure to call this "Mexican Soup" if you want your kids to eat it!*

3 large Eggplants	1 c. Olive Oil
2 large Yellow Onions	6 cloves crushed Garlic
6 c. GF Chicken Broth	6 c. fresh or canned Tomatoes
1 tsp. Ground Cumin	2 tsp. Dried Oregano
1 tsp. Sea Salt	1 tsp. Pepper
Juice of 1 Lemon	

Slice eggplant into ½-inch strips; grill or broil until tender. Cool slightly and cut in chunks. In a large stockpot combine olive oil, onion, and garlic; sauté until tender about 10 minutes, stirring often. Add eggplant, broth, lemon juice, spices, and tomatoes; cook 5 minutes. Puree in small batches in blender and return to pot. Add more spices if desired.

Sunshine Soup

3 chopped medium Onions	2 chopped Leeks
4 chopped Carrots	2 chopped Turnips
3 chopped Parsnips	1 chopped Rutabaga
4 T. Earth Balance or Grass-fed Butter	1½ quarts GF Chicken Broth
4 Thyme Sprigs	4 cloves minced Garlic

Sea Salt & Pepper	Pinch of Nutmeg

Pinch Cayenne Pepper – *optional*

Melt Earth Balance in stockpot and add onions, leeks, carrots, turnips, rutabaga, and parsnips. Cover and cook for 30 minutes over low heat, stirring occasionally. Add chicken broth and bring to a boil. Add garlic, thyme, and cayenne. Cover and simmer for about 30 minutes until veggies are soft. Remove thyme and puree soup in blender in small batches. Return to pot and ladle into bowls.

BLACK BEAN STEW

1 T. Olive Oil	1 Onion, chopped
2 cloves crushed Garlic	1 tsp. Ground Cumin
2 tsp. GF Taco or Chipotle Seasoning	2 c. GF Organic Chicken Broth
1 can Black Beans	1-2 tsp. Sea Salt
½ c. frozen Organic Corn	½ c. diced Tomatoes
½ c. Fresh Cilantro	Tofutti Sour Cream
Brown Rice	

Cook rice according to package directions. Heat oil on medium heat in a large pot. Add onion, garlic, cumin, and Mexican seasoning. Sauté until onions are tender. Add beans, broth, and spices. Raise the heat and bring to a boil. Reduce heat and simmer covered for at least 1 hour. Salt to taste. Add corn, tomatoes, and cilantro. Serve over cooked rice and top with Tofutti sour cream if desired.

CHICKEN BROWN RICE SOUP

2 c. Raw Brown Rice

Sea Salt & Pepper

3 Celery, chopped

4 Organic Potatoes, cubed

2 boxes Organic Chicken Broth

2 Chicken Breasts, cubed

3 Carrots, chopped

1 large Onion, chopped

4 cloves crushed Garlic

Place the chicken breasts in a stockpot and cover them with water. Boil until chicken is fully cooked. Remove chicken and dice into bite size pieces. Pour broth into water. Season with salt and pepper. Add carrots, celery, onion, potato, and garlic. Add rice. Return chicken and simmer until veggies and rice are tender (For quick preparation, boil veggies until tender.) Season with salt and pepper to taste.

ENCHILADA SOUP

2 large Skinless Boneless
  Chicken Breast

1 c. GF Salsa

1 (14.5 oz.) Tomato Sauce

Tofutti Sour Cream

2 (15 oz) cans Diced
  Tomatoes or fresh

1 (4oz) can Green Chilies

2 (15 oz) cans Black Beans

Organic Corn Chips

Goat Gouda or Cheddar (Rice or Soy: Cheddar) *optional*

Place all ingredients into crock-pot and cook on low for 8 hours. Just before serving take out chicken, shred, and return to soup. Serve topped with cheese of choice, Tofutti sour cream, and dip with organic corn chips.

NOTES

VEGETABLE RECIPES

GREEN BEAN & RED PEPPER SAUTÉ

1 bag frozen or 2 handfuls
  cleaned Green Beans

Olive Oil

1 Organic Red Pepper,
  cleaned & sliced very thin

Garlic Salt & Pepper

In a sauté pan, slowly heat a thin layer of olive oil on medium heat. Toss in peppers and green beans. Season with garlic salt and pepper. Cook until beans reach desired tenderness. (For well done "squishy" beans like my kids will eat, I cover the pan and cook them until squishy.)

SPINACH, TOMATOES, & GOAT CHEESE

◆ *This can't be done 100% Dairy-Free*

1 bunch fresh Spinach
  or 1 bag frozen Spinach

½ to 1 container Grape
  Tomatoes

1 container crumbled
  Goat Feta Cheese

Olive Oil

Put a layer of olive oil into a sauté pan. Set on low heat. Put spinach in pan and cover until wilted – just a few minutes – watch carefully. Toss in tomatoes for a brief moment (they heat up quickly, too). Put in a bowl and add feta, tossing to mix. Serve immediately!

BLACK BEANS

Olive Oil

½ c. finely diced Onion

½ tsp. minced Garlic

2 (15 oz.) cans Black Beans

¼ tsp. Sea Salt

½ c. chopped Grape Tomatoes

2 T. diced fresh Cilantro

Heat a layer of oil in a large sauté pan, on medium heat. Sauté onion until transparent. Add garlic and sauté a minute or two. Stir in black beans (rinsed and drained) and sea salt. Cook until heated through. Stir in grape tomatoes and fresh cilantro. *(More than 2 T. cilantro is great, too. You can never have too much cilantro and it's a great detoxifier for your body as well!)* Serve immediately.

GRILLED VEGGIES

4 Organic Red Potatoes

1 large Zucchini

1 Bell Pepper – *we like red best*

½ lb. Asparagus

1 medium Red Onion, sliced

Lay out a large piece of tin foil. Cover foil with an equal size piece of parchment paper to protect your food from absorbing harmful aluminum toxins. Chop up the vegetables and place on top of the parchment paper. Drizzle generously with olive oil, sea salt, and pepper. Close foil making sure none of veggies are touching foil but are protected by parchment paper. Place on grill over medium heat and let cook about 10 minutes, flip and continue to grill for another 10-15 minutes until veggies are tender.

POTATO SALAD

5 Organic Potatoes diced to bite size	3 hard boiled Eggs
½ cup chopped Onion	½ c. GF Pickles
¼ T. Garlic Salt	¼ T. Celery Salt
1 T. GF Mustard	¼ c. Spectrum Canola Mayo
Ground Black Pepper to taste	

HOMEMADE GF BAKED BEANS

6 slices Turkey Bacon	1 c. chopped Onion
1 clove minced Garlic	¾ c. GF Ketchup
16 oz. can Pinto Beans w/ juice	16 oz. can Great Northern Beans, drained
2 (16oz.) cans Black Beans w/juice	16 oz. can Red Kidney Beans, drained
½ c. Molasses	¼ c. Organic Brown Sugar
2 T. GF BBQ Sauce	1 T. GF Mustard
½ tsp. Pepper	

Preheat oven to 375. Cook bacon, remove from pan, add oil if needed; sauté onion and garlic until onion is tender. In a 9 x 13 pan or casserole dish, mix ketchup, molasses, brown sugar, BBQ sauce, mustard, and pepper. Then add beans, stir well, cover and bake for about 1 hour.

ROASTED BABY RED POTATOES
w/ROSEMARY & GARLIC

12-14 Baby Red Potatoes,
  cut in quarters

2 large cloves Garlic,
  chopped coarsely

1 T. fresh Rosemary

1 T. Olive Oil (or more)

1 tsp. Sea Salt

Pepper to taste

Preheat oven to 350 degrees. Place potatoes in 9 x 13 pan. Drizzle with olive oil. Evenly sprinkle with rosemary, garlic, salt, and pepper. Place in oven. Roast until outsides are crisp, brown, and easily pierced with a fork.

ARTICHOKES

PAN METHOD: Place artichokes in a saucepan with 1½ to 2 inches of water in it. Cover and cook for 45-50 minutes. Make sure to check water often to make sure you do not burn the pan by running out of water.

STEAMER METHOD: Prepare steamer and steam artichokes for about 50 minutes to 1 hour.

WINTER SQUASH

1 Winter Squash – *any variety*

4 T. EB or Grass-fed Butter

Cut squash in half. Clean seeds out and place skin side down on a shallow baking sheet. Place 2 T. Earth Balance in each squash half. Bake in a 350-degree oven for about 60 minutes until tender when poked with a fork.

ROASTED ASPARAGUS

1 lb Asparagus   2 T. Olive Oil

Sea Salt   ¼ c. Pecorino Cheese

Cut bottoms off asparagus and wash. Place asparagus in a 9 x 13 pan. Drizzle olive oil over asparagus, sprinkle with sea salt and toss. Bake for about 10 minutes in a 350-degree oven until bright green. Serve with pecorino cheese sprinkled on top.

GARLIC MASHED POTATOES

6 Potatoes (peeled & boiled)   1 T. crushed Garlic

½ stick of EB or Grass-fed   ¼ c. or more Rice/Almond
  Butter   Milk

1 tsp. Onion Powder   Sea Salt & Pepper to taste

Place cooked potatoes, butter, garlic, milk and onion powder in a mixer. Mix until smooth. Add milk until you find the texture you like for mashed potatoes, then add salt and pepper to taste.

AUNT TOODLE'S VEGGIE DIP

1 c. Tofutti Sour Cream   1 c. Spectrum Canola Mayo

1 tsp. Dill Weed   1 tsp. Parsley Flakes

1-2 tsp. diced Onion   1 tsp. Garlic Salt

Mix all ingredients and refrigerate in a sealed container. It will keep for up to one week.

ROASTED CAULIFLOWER W/BROWNED BUTTER

1 head of Cauliflower   Olive Oil Cooking Spray

¼ tsp. Sea Salt   ¼ tsp. Pepper

2 tsp. EB or Grass-fed Butter

Preheat oven to 400 degrees. Arrange cauliflower florets in a single layer on a baking sheet. Coat with a light layer of olive oil spray, sprinkle with sea salt and pepper. Bake for 25 minutes, turning twice. Melt Earth Balance in a sauce pan over medium heat, and cook until lightly browned, about three minutes. (Be careful because it burns easily!) Place roasted cauliflower in large bowl, pour butter over it and toss gently to coat.

MASHED CAULIFLOWER

1 head of Cauliflower   Dash of Rice Milk

1 T. Earth Balance or Grass-   Pinch of Sea Salt & Pepper
fed Butter

Steam cauliflower until soft. Place in food processor. Add Earth Balance, rice milk, salt, and pepper. Puree, adding rice milk as needed to create a mashed potato consistency.

VARIATION: add ½ cup or more of grated Pecorino Romano cheese (sheep) or a sprinkle or two of Nutritional Yeast into puree and then top each serving with a sprinkle of grated cheese.

TWICE BAKED CARROT POTATOES

4 Potatoes   2 Large Carrots

Dash of Milk – *I use rice milk*

Bake the potatoes and slice and boil the carrots. When potatoes are done, cut them in half and scoop the flesh into a medium mixing bowl. Place cooked carrots in the bowl with the potatoes. Add a dash of milk of your choice and whip with hand mixer until smooth. Spoon mixture back into potato skins and place on a cookie sheet. Place in 350-degree oven for about 15 minutes until slightly crunchy on top.

BASIL & BALSAMIC DRESSING

1 c. Olive Oil   ¼ c. Balsamic Vinegar

2 cloves crushed Garlic   ½ tsp. Sea Salt

1 large bunch fresh Basil   1 T. Honey
  Leaves

Place olive oil, vinegar, garlic, sea salt and honey in blender. Blend until well mixed. Add basil leaves and puree. Store in a glass jar in refrigerator until ready to use. Use the same day or freeze unused portions

BALSAMIC VINEGAR & OLIVE OIL

Drizzle balsamic vinegar and olive oil over a romaine or leafy lettuce salad. Add favorite diced veggies and sprinkle with goat crumbles, ground flax, nutritional yeast, etc.

Basil-Infused Olive Oil & Balsamic Vinegar

Drizzle basil-infused olive oil and balsamic vinegar over a romaine or leafy lettuce salad. Sprinkle with Gorgonzola cheese or goat crumbles if desired.

My Kids' Favorite Italian Dressing

1 c. Olive Oil	⅓ c. Red Wine Vinegar
4 cloves fresh crushed Garlic (or 4 tsp. crushed)	1 tsp. Sea Salt
⅔ tsp. Dry Ground Mustard	1 tsp. Oregano
¼ small Red Onion, diced very fine	

Place all ingredients in a container with a tight fitting lid. Cover and shake vigorously! Let sit for a while to blend flavors. Prepare individual salads (romaine lettuce is best), spoon desired amount of dressing over each salad, sprinkle Gorgonzola cheese over each, and enjoy! Dressing lasts up to one week in cupboard.

Our Favorite Salad Toppings

•Kalamata Olives	•Diced Carrot Bites
•Avocado Chunks	•Cilantro – diced
•Scallions – the green part	•Grape Tomatoes
•Blue Cheese – occasionally	•Red Onion Slices – very thin

Auntie Anne's Watermelon Greek Salad

2 tsp. diced fresh Mint

1 tsp. Lime Juice

1 handful diced Italian
Parsley

2 c. chopped Watermelon

1 container Goat Feta Cheese

½–1 c. diced Black Olives

1 small Red Onion, finely diced

Toss all ingredients in bowl. Serve cold. Omit feta for 100% dairy-free.

Raspberry Salad

Great w/Spinach Leaves

2 T. GF Raspberry Vinegar

⅓ c. Olive Oil

2 T. Fruit-Sweetened Raspberry Jam

1 small container Organic
Raspberries

2 Kiwi Fruit

1 bunch fresh Spinach

¾ c. Macadamia Nuts

Mix the raspberry vinegar, olive oil and raspberry jam in a container and shake vigorously.

Peel and slice kiwi fruit. Wash one container of organic raspberries and chop ¾ c. macadamia nuts. Place washed and cleaned spinach in a bowl, top with kiwi, raspberries, and nuts. Add dressing, toss and enjoy.

NOTES

SNACK RECIPES

TACO DIP

6 oz. Tofutti Sour Cream	1 diced small Yellow Onion
2 Ripe Avocados	1 diced Tomato
1 T. Garlic Salt	Chopped Romaine Lettuce
1 T. Ground Cumin	

On a large plate or small platter, smear the Tofutti sour cream. Cut the avocados in half and scoop into a bowl. Mash with fork until smooth. Stir in 1 T. garlic salt. Spread this over the sour cream. Dice the onion very fine (you should have about 2½ T.). Sprinkle on top of avocados. Tear or cut romaine lettuce into bite-size pieces. Sprinkle liberally over avocados. Dice the tomato and sprinkle over lettuce. Serve with organic corn chips.

BEAN DIP

2 cans (15.5 oz.) Organic Pinto Beans	1 c. shredded Goat Gouda (Rice/Soy: Cheddar)
½ c. GF Salsa	Organic Corn Tortilla Chips

Place beans in a small saucepan and cook over medium heat; as you heat the beans, mash them with a fork until they are smooth. When heated through, add cheese and salsa. Heat for one minute and serve with organic corn chips.

Jeanne's Peanut Dip

⅔ c. Organic Creamy Peanut   ¼ c. Honey or Maple Syrup
  Butter

⅓ c. Brown Rice Vinegar   3 T. Water

2 T. GF Tamari Soy Sauce   1 T. fresh minced Ginger

2 cloves crushed Garlic   1½ tsp. Toasted Sesame Oil

¼ tsp. crushed Red Pepper   1 c. chopped fresh Cilantro
  Flakes – *optional*   (packed loosely)

Blend all ingredients except cilantro until smooth. Add cilantro and pulse briefly until just chopped. Serve with any veggies, especially red peppers. It is also awesome with fried tofu.

Guacamole

6 Avocados   1 Lime

1 T. Spectrum Canola Mayo   Garlic Salt to taste

Organic Corn Chips

Clean avocados, cut in half and scoop flesh into a mixing bowl. Mash with a fork until smooth. Add mayo, the juice of half a lime and garlic salt to taste (start with 1 tsp., then taste with chip and continue to add garlic salt until you like the taste). Stir well. To preserve guacamole, retain the avocado pit and keep it in the container of guacamole, or put a slice of lime on top to preserve and keep it from browning.

KELLI'S GLUTEN-FREE CHEWY GRANOLA BARS

½ c. EB (cut in cubes)
  or Grass-fed Butter

½ c. Gluten-Free/Dairy-Free
  Chocolate Chips

⅓ c. Organic Brown Sugar

¼ c. Brown Rice Flour

1 tsp. Baking Soda

½ c. finely chopped Pecans

½ c. Currants

½ c. Rice Bran

½ c. Sunflower Seeds

½ c. Honey

½ c. Dried Apricots

4½ c. GF Rolled Oats

Preheat oven to 350 degrees and butter (or spray with olive oil) a 9 x 13 pan. In a large bowl mix oats, brown sugar, flour, and baking soda. Then add pecans, currants, chocolate chips, sunflower seeds and rice bran and set aside. Place apricots in a small food processor and process until smooth. Add Earth Balance and process again until smooth. With food processor running, add honey through the feeding tube and process until smooth. Fold apricot mixture into oat mixture. Press firmly into pan until level. Place in oven, bake about 30 minutes, until golden brown. Put pan on wire rack and allow to cool *completely!* Cut into bars and remove from pan. Wrap each bar in wax paper and then plastic. Store in airtight container or freeze.

◆FOR DAIRY-FREE: *substitute coconut oil or dairy-free butter, your choice.*

BANA-CICLES

Peel bananas. Place a Popsicle stick in the bottom of each banana. Place in a large Ziploc bag and freeze overnight.

SHELBY'S GRANOLA BARS

3½ c. Oats	¾ c. Raisins
⅔ c. Sunflower Seeds	½ c. Toasted Sesame Seeds
½ c. Wheat Germ	½ c. Oat Bran
1 T. Cinnamon	1 tsp. Sea Salt
1 c. Organic Coconut	1 c. Honey
1 c. chopped Organic Almonds	1-2 c. GF/DF Chocolate Chips
5 T. Grass-fed Butter	1½ c. Organic Creamy Peanut Butter

3 T. Flax Seeds or Ground Flax

In a large bowl combine oats, sunflower seeds, chocolate chips, wheat germ, salt, raisins, sesame seeds, oat bran, cinnamon, coconut, and almonds. In a pan melt butter and peanut butter. Remove from heat and add honey. Pour into dry mix and mix well. Press into a 9 x 13 (buttered) pan. Bake in a 350-degree oven for 15 minutes. Cut in desired sizes, wrap in plastic wrap and store in refrigerator.

FROZEN CHOCOLATE BANANAS

3 large Bananas	1 c. GF/DF Chocolate Chips
1 T. Grass-fed Butter	½ c. chopped Nuts (of choice)

Peel bananas and cut them in half. Push Popsicle stick halfway into banana. Freeze overnight in a Ziplock bag. Melt chocolate chips and butter in a saucepan. Dip bananas in melted chocolate and then roll in chopped nuts.

DOG BONES

½ c. Organic Peanut Butter

1 T. Honey

2 T. GF Graham Cracker Crumbs

1 tsp. Ground Flax

½ c. Dairy-Free Powder, Powdered Milk or Powdered Coconut Milk

In a bowl mix peanut butter, flax, dry dairy-free or powdered. Add honey and mix very well. Divide dough into 6 pieces and mold into bone shapes – or any shape you would like. Sprinkle both sides with graham crackers.

SHELBY'S COWBOY CAVIAR

1 can Black-Eyed Peas

1 can Shoepeg Corn

⅔ c. chopped Cilantro

⅔ c. chopped Green Onion

1 Avocado, diced

1 Roma Tomato, diced

DRESSING:

¼ c. Olive Oil

¼ c. Red Wine Vinegar

1+ tsp. Garlic, crushed

1 tsp. Ground Cumin

¾ tsp. Sea Salt

¼ tsp. Pepper

Place all veggies into a large bowl. Mix dressing ingredients in a small bowl and pour onto veggie mix. Serve with organic corn chips.

GRANOLA BARS

3½ c. GF Oats   ¾ c. Raisins

⅔ c. Sunflower Seeds   ½ c. Brown Rice Flour

½ c. Rice Bran   3 T. Ground Flaxseeds

1 T. Cinnamon   1 tsp. Sea Salt

1 c. Shredded Coconut   1 c. Almonds (chopped fine)

1 c. Honey   5 T. EB or Grass-fed Butter

1½ c. Organic Creamy Peanut Butter

1 c. Enjoy Life (GF/DF) Chocolate Chips (if desired). SunDrops by SunSpire are really good as well. They're like M&Ms but don't have food coloring or HFCS.

In a large bowl combine: oats, sunflower seeds, rice bran, cinnamon, coconut, raisins, flour, flax, sea salt and almonds. In a different bowl stir peanut butter, honey, and melted Earth Balance together. Pour mixture over dry ingredients and mix well. Press into a foil/parchment lined 9 x 13 pan. Bake in a 350-degree oven for about 15 minutes. Remove from oven, sprinkle chocolate chips over top (or you can mix them in, depending on how you like your bars – topped with chocolate or mixed in) and return to oven for about 2 minutes. Refrigerate until firm. Cut, and wrap individually. Store in refrigerator and they freeze well.

TRAIL MIX
THAT FEEDS MY BRAIN & KEEPS ME HEALTHY!

1 c. dried Blueberries   1 c. dried Cranberries

1 c. Sunflower Seeds   ½ c. Peanuts

½ c. SunDrop Candies
  (by SunSpire)

Place all ingredients in a bowl. Toss and eat!

◆Blueberries and cranberries are high in antioxidants and boost the immune system to keep you strong and healthy! The nuts and seeds are great for nourishing your brain with good fats. Did you know 80% of your brain is made from fat? The crunch helps to alert your brain and keep you focused, so this is a good snack for homework time. The SunDrops are naturally sweetened with evaporated cane juice (better than refined sugar) and are colored with veggies like beets, not artificial colors and dyes. SunDrops also have buttermilk in them, which is another good source of healthy fat to feed our brains. Not only will you enjoy eating this snack, it actually will help you to be healthier and smarter!

SOUR CREAM/SALSA MEXICAN CHIP DIP

½ c. Tofutti Sour Cream   Corn Chips

1 c. Salsa – Homemade or store bought

Mix sour cream and salsa together; use as a chip dip.

3-PEPPER BRUSCHETTA

1 pack Mini Belle Sweet
Pepper Mix

1 medium Purple Onion,
sliced thin (or ½ red,
½ yellow, ½ orange peppers)

Sea Salt & Pepper to taste

1 T. fresh minced basil,
sliced thin

12 slices of GF Baguette
(I use hot dog buns cut
into disks)

2 T. Olive Oil

Brush each circle of bread on one side with olive oil, place in 350-degree oven and toast until golden brown. Remove from oven. Heat a skillet with olive oil in it, add peppers and onion; sauté until tender. Remove from heat and cool slightly. Toss basil, salt and pepper into pepper mixture. Top each piece of bread with pepper mixture and bake for about 5 minutes to heat through, serve immediately!

BRUSCHETTA

DICE THE FOLLOWING VERY FINE:

1 peeled Cucumber

1 big handful of Basil

1 dry pint of Organic Mini
Sweet Peppers

Sea Salt & Pepper to taste

2-3 cloves crushed Garlic

1 small Purple Onion

1 big handful of Parsley

Juice from 1 Organic
Lemon

1 T. Olive Oil

Dice, place in a bowl, and mix well. Serve on crostini, GF crackers, or organic corn chips. Crostini: Sliced GF French bread brushed with olive oil and toasted in a 425-degree oven.

HUMMUS

2 c. Chickpeas – drained or
  well rinsed if canned

½ c. fresh Lemon Juice
  (freshly squeezed organic)

3 Garlic cloves, crushed

1 c. Tahini

½ tsp. Sea Salt

½-1 c. Water

Food Processor

Combine chickpeas and garlic in food processor. Add lemon juice, tahini, salt, and 1/2 c. water. Process until very smooth and creamy. At least 2 minutes! Should be consistency of mashed potatoes. If thick and pasty, add water with the food processor running until it's smooth and creamy.

Serve with corn chips; rice crackers, or fresh raw veggies. Or use as a spread for sandwiches.

MEAT, CHEESE & CRACKER RING

Various nitrate/nitrite-free meats:
Salami, Ham, Pepperoni, Turkey, etc.

Various GF Crackers

Various Cheeses:
Goat Gouda, Goat Herb Roll, etc.

Slice various meats and cheese and place on a plate. Place crackers in a ring around the edge of plate and let them dig in.

JUICE POPSICLES

◆Great affordable alternative to popsicles filled with food coloring and sugar!

100% Juice of your choice	1 or more ice cube trays
Aluminum Foil	Toothpicks

Fill ice cube trays ¾ full with juice and place aluminum foil over tray. *Foil should not touch juice since cubes aren't frozen.* Place 1 toothpick through foil into each cube. (The foil keeps the toothpick in place.) Place in freezer overnight. Remove foil immediately, pop out cubes with toothpicks frozen into them and place in a large resealable bag; return to freezer.

◆You can also make a smoothie and freeze it, as you would juice, for a variation on the popsicles.

HOMEMADE SALSA & CORN CHIPS

10 Tomatoes	1 large Red Pepper
¾ small Green Pepper	4 slices of a Jalapeño
3 tsp. Salt	3 tsp. Pepper
3 tsp. Lemon Juice	1 clove chopped Garlic
¼ small Purple Onion	Cilantro – to taste
Food Processor	Corn Chips

Clean vegetables. Put everything except tomatoes in food processor and blend. Add tomatoes to taste and serve with corn chips.

VARIATIONS: For a spicier salsa, add banana peppers and more jalapenos. For a milder salsa add more tomatoes.

CRACKER STACKERS

GF Crackers

PIZZA:

Pizza Sauce (page 163)   Goat Cheese

Pepperoni   Canadian Bacon

Layer pizza sauce and toppings, then heat in oven or microwave.

JAMMIN':

Tofutti Cream Cheese   Polaner All-Fruit Jam

Layer cream cheese and jam.

VEGETABLES:

Tomatoes   Basil

Olive Oil   Salt & Pepper

Dice tomatoes and basil. Toss with olive oil. Salt and pepper to taste.

Toast GF bagels in oven and serve veggie mix on top of hot bagels.
Great with a dash of goat cheese on top, too.

LETTUCE PEANUT BUTTER WRAPS

Leaf Lettuce (or Romaine)   Organic Peanut Butter
  not Iceburg!   No Sugar

Wash lettuce. Spread peanut butter on lettuce. Roll and eat

BUTTERLESS POPCORN

Organic Popcorn   Coconut Oil – *great flavor!*

Sea Salt

Heat up coconut oil in a heavy and deep pan. Add popcorn kernels. Heat, shaking as necessary as not to burn. Serve with sea salt sprinkled over top. If you would like butter, just melt some grass-fed butter or Earth Balance and drizzle it over the top.

TACO DIP

1 Tomato   Leaf or Romaine Lettuce

1/4 small Onion,   2-3 Avocados
  diced very small

Garlic Salt   Canola Mayo (Spectrum)

8 oz. Tofutti Cream Cheese   8 oz. Tofutti Sour Cream

Blend sour cream with cream cheese. Spread on a dinner-size plate. Clean out and mash avocados. Add garlic salt to taste and 1 T. of mayo. Spread this mixture over cream cheese mixture. Sprinkle onion over avocado. Shred lettuce and spread over onion layer. Top with diced tomato.

VARIATION: Add taco seasoning to the sour cream mixture to add a little zip. Serve with salsa on the side.

JAYNE'S BEAN DIP

2 Tomatoes	2 cans Shoepeg Corn
1 Avocado	2 cans Black Beans
1 Purple Onion, diced fine	Garlic Salt to taste
1 Lime	Corn Chips

Clean and dice vegetables, then toss them in a bowl – mix well. Add garlic salt to taste. Squeeze in lime juice and mix, to prevent browning of avocado.

Mix a dollop of sour cream with some salsa to make a pink color. The more sour cream the less spicy the salsa – alter to taste. Serve with corn chips.

ANTS ON A LOG

Celery & Raisins	Peanut Butter – no sugar

Clean and cut celery into sticks. Spread peanut butter on each celery stick. Place a few raisins on each peanut butter filled celery stick.

FRUIT w/PEANUT BUTTER

Organic Peanut Butter *– no sugar*	Apples or Bananas

Place peanut butter in a bowl for each child. Give them apple slices or a banana and let them dip and eat.

WINGS

1 c. Tamari GF Soy Sauce   2 cloves Garlic

Chicken Wings

Marinate chicken wings in soy sauce and garlic for a few hours, doesn't need to be overnight. Bake in oven at 350 degrees until cooked through, or all day in crock-pot for an after school snack.

BUTTERFLY TREATS

3 stalks of Celery   12 GF Pretzel Twists

GF Pretzel Pieces   Raisins or Currants

6 T. Sun Butter or Peanut Butter

Cut celery in half crosswise. Fill each piece of celery with 1 T. peanut butter or sun butter. Add 2 pretzel wings. Use pieces of pretzels for antennae and raisins/currants for decoration.

PEANUT BUTTER TORTILLAS

GF Tortillas   Organic Peanut Butter
                                          – *no sugar*

Polaner All Fruit – Jelly/Jam or Fruit Juice-Sweetened Jam, Honey or Agave Nectar

Spread peanut butter (and jelly if desired) over tortilla. Roll. Eat! Great for picnics and lunch boxes!

POTATO SKINS

3 Potatoes

½-1 c. Tofutti Sour Cream

Sea Salt & Pepper

3 T. Chives

Dash Rice Milk

Pecorino Cheese

Bake potatoes in oven at 425 degrees for about 1 hour or until tender. Cut each potato in half and scoop insides into a bowl. Mash potato. Dice up chives and add to potatoes. Add sour cream to desired texture. Thin with rice milk if needed. Add salt and pepper to taste. Spoon back into each potato skin shell and top with pecorino cheese. Return to oven and bake until golden brown.

STUFFED EGGS

3 Hard Boiled Eggs

¼ tsp. Sea Salt

Dash of Pepper

2 T. Spectrum Canola Mayo

Black Olives – cut in half

⅛ tsp. Ground Cumin

Peel cooled eggs. Cut in half and scoop out yolks. Use a fork to mash yolks in a small bowl. Add mayo, sea salt, cumin, and pepper – stir well. Fill each egg with yolk mixture and top with half an olive. Chill and eat.

Frozen Fruits & Veggies

For snack foods, my kids really enjoy frozen fruits and veggies. They love frozen blueberries, mixed berries, peaches, peas, and green beans. We also juice beets and Granny Smith apples (1 beet to 3 apples) and freeze them as popsicles.

PICKLE ROLL UPS

GF Pickles   Ham slices or Turkey
  (nitrite/sulfite-free)   (nitrite/sulfite-free)

Tofutti Cream Cheese

Spread cream cheese on a piece of ham. Place a pickle on the ham. Roll. Slice into ¼ to ½-inch bite-size pieces.

Bread & Dip

GF Bread (sliced Hot Dog   Balsamic Vinegar (*if desired*
  Buns or a Baguette)   *for some spice*)

Olive Oil   Grated Pecorino Cheese

Place olive oil and pecorino cheese, mixed on a plate. (If desired, add balsamic.) Dip bread and eat!

Rice Cakes w/Peanut or Sun Butter

Rice Cakes (Brown Rice)   Organic Peanut Butter
                                     or Sun Butter

Spread peanut butter on rice cake and add Honey, Agave or Fruit Juice-Sweetened Jam.

TRAIL MIX

Nuts of all varieties   Raisins

GF/DF Chocolate Chips or   Dried Fruit of choice
   SunDrops *(they do have dairy)*

Toss whatever you would like in a bowl and eat. My kids love to make their own mixtures for a snack.

SMOOTHIE ICE CREAM

Use any recipe from the smoothie section.

Make smoothie, place in cups and put in freezer until solid.

Eat with a spoon.

NOTES

NATURALLY SWEETENED OR LOW SUGAR
DESSERT RECIPES

◆Use Earth Balance STICKS for all baking – do not use whipped! Or use grass-fed butter.

HAWAIIAN CREAM CHEESE FROSTING

8 oz. Tofutti Cream Cheese

¼ c. Xylitol

1 T. Pineapple Juice
  (from canned pineapple)

4 T. Coconut Oil

1 tsp. GF Vanilla

2 T. Grated Coconut

Cream together the coconut oil and cream cheese until smooth. Mix in the xylitol, pineapple juice, grated coconut and vanilla until well blended. Frost cooled cake.

CREAM CHEESE FROSTING
DAIRY-FREE NATURALLY SWEETENED

8 oz. Tofutti Cream Cheese

¼ c. Xylitol

4 T. EB or Grass-fed Butter

1 tsp. GF Vanilla

Cream the Earth Balance and cream cheese together until smooth. Add Xylitol and cream. Add vanilla until well blended. Frost cooled cake.

✔ HEAD START TIP: *These frostings freeze really well.*

CARROT CAKE

1½ c. Earth Balance

1¾ c. Xylitol or Raw Sugar

4 Organic Eggs

3 tsp. GF Vanilla

1 tsp. Organic Lemon Zest

2 c. Brown Rice Flour

2 c. Millet Flour

1 tsp. Xanthan Gum

1 tsp. Sea Salt

½ tsp. Baking Soda

1 T. Baking Powder

1 tsp. Allspice

2 tsp. Cinnamon

2 ½ c. finely shredded
   Carrots (packed)

¼ c. fresh squeezed Organic
   Lemon Juice

Preheat oven to 350 degrees. Spray 9 x 13 pan with olive oil spray. Beat Earth Balance with egg, one at a time. Whip until fluffy. Stir in vanilla and lemon rind. In a separate bowl mix flours, xanthan gum, salt, baking soda, baking powder, allspice, and cinnamon. Toss shredded carrots in lemon juice. Add dry ingredients to egg mixture, alternating with carrots until moist – DO NOT OVER MIX. Spread batter in pan and bake 40-50 minutes or until toothpick comes out clean when poked in the center.

◆Great plain, or top with cream cheese frosting

APPLE CRISP

8 medium, peeled and sliced
  Apples

1 T. Cinnamon

1¼ c. Brown Rice Flour

¾ c. Earth Balance, melted

½ tsp. Baking Powder

1 c. Honey, divided

1 c. Almond Meal

½ tsp. Sea Salt

⅛ tsp. Baking Soda

GLUTEN-FREE PUMPKIN BARS/CAKE

1 c. Olive Oil

2 c. canned/fresh Pumpkin

2 c. Gluten-Free Flour Mix
  (see below)

2 tsp. Baking Powder

½ tsp. Sea Salt

4 Organic Eggs

1 c. Xylitol or Raw Sugar

1 tsp. Baking Soda

2 (generous) tsp. Cinnamon

GLUTEN-FREE FLOUR MIX: 2 parts brown rice flour, ⅔ parts potato flour/starch, ⅓ part tapioca flour.

Put all ingredients in a bowl and mix until well blended. Divide equally between two 9 x 13 pans sprayed with olive oil. Bake 15-20 minutes in a 350-degree oven (until toothpicks come out clean).

This is great plain or with cream cheese frosting (page 215).

FRENCH SILK PIE

2 c. EB or Grass-fed Butter	¼ c. Xylitol
¼ c. Honey	¼ c. Maple Syrup
½ c. GF/DF Chocolate Chips	2 tsp. Unsweetened Cocoa
2 tsp. GF Vanilla	4 Organic Eggs
One 9-inch GF Pie Crust	

(I use the Bob's Redmill GF Biscuit Mix and follow the recipe for a pie crust.)

Melt chocolate chips and then allow to cool. In a large bowl, cream butter, xylitol, honey, and maple syrup until smooth. Blend in cooled melted chocolate and vanilla. On medium speed, add one egg at a time, beating each one for five minutes. Pour filling into pie shell, sprinkle chocolate chips on top of the pie and chill at least four hours.

NATURALLY SWEETENED CHOCOLATE FROSTING

6 T. Earth Balance (soft)	2 c. Xylitol or Raw Sugar
1 T. Honey	½ c. Unsweetened Cocoa-Powder
2-3 T. Rice Milk	1 tsp. GF Vanilla

Beat Earth Balance and vanilla until creamy. Combine xylitol or raw sugar and cocoa powder in a separate bowl and then slowly add into the butter mixture, alternating with rice milk, until you reach the consistency desired.

Root Beer Floats

◆ *This is a naturally sweetened treat with out dairy or gluten!*

Coconut Vanilla Bean Ice Cream— *so delicious*

Zevia Root Beer Soda

Place one or two scoops of ice cream in a cup. Top with root beer and enjoy! You can also use rice or soy based ice cream. However, the coconut ice cream is sweetened with agave and has great fats for your brain, so it's a better choice.

Snicker Doodle Cookies

½ cup Earth Balance or Grass-fed Butter

¾ cup packed Organic Brown Sugar

1 Egg

1 tsp. GF Vanilla

1 c. Brown Rice Flour

½ cup Tapioca Flour

½ tsp. Cream of Tartar

¼ tsp. Xanthan Gum

½ tsp. Baking Soda

¼ tsp. Sea Salt

Preheat oven to 375 degrees. In a large bowl, mix together flours, xanthan gum, cream of tartar, baking soda, and sea salt; set aside. With an electric mixer, cream together the butter, brown sugar, egg, and pure vanilla. Slowly add dry ingredients into creamed mixture and beat. Roll into balls, place on non-stick cookie sheet and flatten slightly with a fork in a crisscross pattern. Bake for 8-10 minutes.

So Healthy Brownies

6 T. EB or Grass-fed Butter

¼ c. Almond Meal

1 T. Ground Golden Flax

1 T. Unsweetened Cocoa - Powder

¼ c. Honey

¼ c. Pure Maple Syrup

1 c. crushed nuts of any variety (*optional*)

¼ c.+ 2 T. Millet Flour

2 large Organic Eggs

2 tsp. GF Vanilla

¾ cup Semi-Sweet Chocolate Chips

¼ tsp. Sea Salt

½ c. Purple Puree

Purple Puree: 1½ c. blueberries, 3 cups raw or frozen spinach leaves, 1 T. lemon juice, 3-4 T. water. Place all ingredients into a food processor/blender and puree. (Freeze extra puree in ½ cup portions.)

Double the batch for a 9 x 13 pan.

Preheat oven to 350 degrees. Spray an 8 x 8 glass baking dish with olive oil. Melt Earth Balance in a saucepan over low heat. Add chocolate chips and stir continuously until melted. Set aside to cool. In another bowl, blend the eggs, vanilla, honey, maple syrup, and purple puree. In a mixing bowl, combine the millet flour, almond meal, golden flax, cocoa powder, and salt. Pour chocolate chip mixture into wet ingredients. Slowly add dry ingredients, stirring until all lumps are gone, and pour into greased baking dish. Bake for about 25-30 minutes. Insert a toothpick; if it comes out clean they are done!

NATURALLY SWEETENED BROWNIES

3 Organic Eggs	1 c. Xylitol
¼ c. Grass-fed Butter or EB	2 T. Unsweetened Apple-sauce
⅓ c. Cocoa Powder	¼ c. Millet Flour
⅛ tsp. Sea Salt	2 tsp. Vanilla
⅔ c. chopped Pecans *(optional)*	

Butter an 8 x 8 pan. In bowl, beat eggs and xylitol until mixed well. Add melted butter and applesauce; stir well. In a separate bowl, mix cocoa powder, flour, and salt. Combine flour mixture into egg mixture. Stir in vanilla and pecans. Spoon into pan and bake for 25-30 minutes or until toothpick inserted comes out clean.

◆FOR DAIRY FREE: substitute coconut oil or dairy-free butter alternative for butter.

OOEY, GOOEY BROWNIES

3 Organic Eggs	½ c. Agave Nectar
¼ c. Grass-fed Butter or EB	2 T. Unsweetened Apple-sauce
½ c. Maple Syrup	⅓ c. Cocoa Powder
½ c. Millet Flour	⅛ tsp. Sea Salt
2 tsp. Vanilla	⅔ c. chopped Pecans *(optional)*

Butter an 8 x 8 pan. In bowl beat eggs, maple syrup and agave until mixed well. Add melted butter and applesauce; stir well. In a separate bowl, mix cocoa powder, flour, and salt. Combine flour mixture into egg mixture. Stir in vanilla and pecans. Spoon into pan and bake for 25-30 minutes or until toothpick inserted comes out clean. They will be ooey and gooey inside. <u>Do not overcook</u>! Serve this with some vanilla coconut ice cream... YUM!

DELICIOUS CUT-OUT SUGAR COOKIES

2 c. Gluten-Free Flour Mix   1 c. EB or Grass-fed Butter
  (*see recipe below*)

¼ c. Coconut Flour   ½ tsp. Xanthan Gum

¾ c. Raw Sugar   2 Organic Egg Yolks

2 tsp GF Vanilla   ⅛ tsp. Sea Salt

<u>Flour Mix</u>: 3 c. brown rice flour, 2¾ c. sweet rice flour, 2¼ c. cornstarch, 2¼ c. garbanzo bean flour, 2 c. tapioca starch, 1¾ white sorghum flour. Blend flours together. Store in a tightly covered container in a cool dry place.

Preheat oven to 350 degrees. Mix flour, coconut flour, xanthan gum, and salt together. In mixing bowl, cream together the Earth Balance and sugar; continue beating for 5 minutes. With mixer on, add egg yolks one at a time, then vanilla. Continue beating until creamy. Reduce speed and add dry ingredients. Refrigerate in bowl for one hour. Roll out dough to ¼ inch on cornstarch-dusted surface; cut in circles or cookie cutter shapes. Place on cookie sheet lined with parchment paper. Bake 8-12 minutes until edges are lightly browned. Cool on cookie sheet 2 minutes. Remove to cooling racks to cool completely.

HONEY BUTTER COOKIES

1 c. Brown Rice Flour	1½ c. Dark Teff Flour
½ tsp. Sea Salt	1 tsp. Xanthan Gum
½ Pure Maple Syrup	½ c. Honey
1 c. Organic Peanut Butter	½ c. Olive Oil

Preheat oven to 350 degrees. In a mixing bowl, cream together the peanut butter, syrup, honey, and oil. In a separate bowl, mix flours, salt, and xanthan gum. Slowly add dry ingredients to creamed ingredients, stirring until well blended. Form into ½-¾ inch balls. Place on a cookie sheet and slightly flatten with a fork, creating a crisscross pattern on the dough. Bake 15-20 minutes. Remove from cookie sheet and let cool.

CRANBERRY CHOCOLATE CHIP COOKIES

⅔ c. EB or Grass-fed Butter	⅔ c. Organic Brown Sugar
2 Organic Eggs	1½ c. GF Oats
¾ c. Brown Rice Flour	¾ c. Millet Flour
¾ tsp. Xanthan Gum	1 tsp. Baking Soda
½ tsp. Sea Salt	¾ c. Dried Cranberries
⅔ c. GF/DF Chocolate Chip	

Preheat oven to 375 degrees. In mixer, beat butter and sugar; add eggs and mix well. In a separate bowl combine oats, flours, baking soda, xanthan gum, and salt. Add to butter mixture. Stir in cranberries and chocolate chips. Drop teaspoonfuls onto ungreased cookie sheet. Bake for 10-12 minutes or until golden brown. Cool on wire rack.

CUT-OUT COOKIES

1 c. Brown Rice Flour   1½ c. Millet Flour

2 tsp. Xanthan Gum   ¾ c. Raw Sugar

1 c. EB or Grass-fed Butter   1 Egg

1 T. GF Vanilla   1 tsp. Baking Powder

2 tsp. Organic Pear Juice (no sugar added)

Preheat oven to 425 degrees. In mixer bowl, cream together the Earth Balance, sugar, vanilla, egg, and pear juice. In a separate bowl, combine flours, xanthan gum, and baking powder. With electric mixer on, slowly add dry ingredients into mixer bowl. Roll out dough to ¼ inch on rice-flour-dusted surface. Cut out cookies with cookie cutters of your choice. Bake on ungreased cookie sheet for 6-10 minutes, until slightly brown around the edges. Cool on a wire rack.

NATURALLY SWEETENED ALMOND DELIGHT COOKIES

1 c. Almonds – ground to   1 jar Fruit Juice-Sweetened
   meal in food processor   Raspberry Jam

¾ c. Millet   1 t. Xantan Gum

¾ c. Brown Rice Flour   ½ c. GF Oat Flour

2 tsp. Baking Powder   ¼ tsp. Sea Salt

⅓ c. Olive Oil   ⅓ c. Pure Maple Syrup

¼ c. Organic Apple Juice   1 tsp. GF Almond Extract

1 tsp. GF Vanilla

Preheat oven to 375 degrees. Whisk oil, syrup, juice, almond and vanilla extract together. In a separate bowl, mix together ground almonds, flours, baking powder, xanthan gum, and salt. Slowly mix dry ingredients into whisked ingredients. Form into tsp.-sized balls and place on cookie sheet. Make a thumbprint indentation in center of each cookie. Bake 15 minutes or until golden brown. Cool on a wire rack. When cookies are cooled, fill thumbprint with raspberry jam.

SURPRISE COOKIES

¾ c. Millet Flour	¼ c. Almond Meal
¾ c. Brown Rice Flour	1 tsp. Xantan Gum
¼ c. GF Oats	¼ c. Ground Flax
1 tsp. Baking Soda	1 tsp. Sea Salt
1 c. Earth Balance (softened)	½ c. Xylitol or Raw Sugar
½ c. Organic Brown Sugar	1 tsp. GF Vanilla
2 large Organic Eggs	1-2 c. SunDrops

Preheat oven to 350 degrees. In a large bowl, mix together the flours, xanthan gum, flax, oats, almond meal, baking soda, and sea salt. Using an electric mixer, cream together the Earth Balance, xylitol or raw sugar, and brown sugar. While mixer is on, add eggs, then vanilla. Gradually add dry ingredients. (For a denser cookie, you may add additional millet flour a little at a time.) When well mixed, remove from mixer and stir in 1-2 cups of SunDrops. Drop by rounded tablespoon on a cookie sheet and bake for about 10-12 minutes until golden brown. Cool on a wire rack.

CHOCOLATE CAKE

CHOCOLATE MIXTURE:

3 T. Unsweetened Organic Cocoa Powder

1⅔ T. EB or Grass-fed Butter

⅓ c. Xylitol

2 tsp. Prune Puree (put 6-8 prunes in blender with 1-2 T. water and puree)

½ c. Water

In a saucepan, combine all ingredients, cook on low heat, stirring until smooth. Remove from heat and cool.

CAKE:

½ c. Melted EB or Grass-fed Butter

1¾ c. Xylitol or Raw Sugar

1¼ c. Brown Rice Flour

1 c. Tapioca Flour

¼ tsp. Xanthan Gum

2 tsp. Baking Soda

½ tsp. Sea Salt

¼ c. Prune Puree

¾ c. Tofutti Sour Cream

1 tsp. GF Vanilla

4 Organic Eggs (separated)

FOR CAKE:

Mixture 1: In a large bowl, combine brown rice flour, tapioca flour, xanthan gum, baking soda, and sea salt; set aside.

Mixture 2: Mix together the melted Earth Balance, egg yolks, vanilla, Tofutti sour cream, and prune puree.

Mixture 3: Using an electric mixer, beat egg whites until soft peaks form. Slowly add xylitol or raw sugar and continue beating until stiff peaks form.

Gradually fold dry ingredients (mixture 1) into beaten egg whites (mixture 3), alternating with the liquid mixture (mixture 2). Do not over stir! When mixed, pour into a greased bundt or 9 x 13 pan. Bake at 350 degrees for about 30 minutes, until toothpick inserted comes out clean.

KELLI'S GLUTEN-FREE CHOCOLATE CHIP COOKIES

1 c. Millet Flour

1 tsp. Baking Soda

1 c. Brown Rice Flour

4½ T. Organic Corn Flour

1 c. Earth Balance (soft)
  or Grass-fed Butter

½-1 c. GF/DF Chocolate
  Chips

½ c. Organic Brown Sugar

½ tsp. Xanthan Gum

2 Organic Eggs

2 tsp. GF Vanilla

½ c. Raw Sugar

1 tsp. Sea Salt

Preheat oven to 375 degrees. Allow Earth Balance to soften. In a small bowl, mix together the flours, baking soda, salt, and xanthan gum. Set aside. Using an electric mixer, cream the Earth Balance and both sugars. Beat in eggs and vanilla. Add dry ingredients and mix on low speed. Stir in chocolate chips. Drop batter by rounded teaspoons onto cookie sheet, spacing then two inches apart. Bake for 12-14 minutes or until golden brown.

HIGH PROTEIN BEANIE COOKIES

½ c. Millet Flour

¼ c. GF Rolled Oats, finely ground

2 T. Almond Meal

¼ c. Organic Brown Sugar

1 Organic Egg

¼ c. White Bean Puree

½ c. Brown Rice Flour

½ tsp. Baking Soda

½ c. GF/DF Chocolate Chips

½ tsp. Sea Salt

¼ tsp. Xanthan Gum

1 tsp. GF Vanilla

¼ c. Raw Sugar

8 T. EB or Grass-fed Butter

WHITE BEAN PUREE:

1 can (15.5 oz.) Organic White Beans (Garbanzo work great)

Put entire can of beans with juices in the bowl of your food processor or in your blender. Puree until mixture is smooth.

Preheat oven to 375 degrees. Allow Earth Balance to soften. In a small bowl, mix together the flour, baking soda, salt, ground oats, gum, and almond meal. Set aside. Using an electric mixer, cream the Earth Balance and both sugars. Beat in egg, vanilla, and white bean puree. Add dry ingredients and mix on low speed. Stir in chocolate chips. Make bite-size cookies by dropping rounded ½ tsp. of batter, spaced 2 inches apart, onto a cookie sheet. Bake for 12-14 minutes or until golden brown.

◆*For a denser cookie add more millet flour.*

Nutty Bars

2 c. Organic Peanut Butter	1 c. Honey
2 c. Raw Brown Sesame Seeds	1 c. Sunflower Seeds
½ c. crushed Cashews	¼-½ c. shaved Coconut

In a large bowl, mix honey and peanut butter. Stir in the sesame seeds. Mix in the sunflower seeds. Add the cashews and mix. Add the coconut and make sure all ingredients are thoroughly combined.

Adjust flavors:

If too dry, add more peanut butter	If too salty, add a touch more honey
If bland, add more coconut	If too moist, add sesame seeds

Press mixture into an 8 x 8 pan (for thick bars) or 9 x 13 pan (for thinner bars). Refrigerate until firm. Cut to size. You can wrap them tightly in plastic wrap for transport. Keep stored in the refrigerator.

Layer the apple slices on the bottom of 9 x 13 pan. Drizzle 1/2 cup of honey and sprinkle the cinnamon over the apples. In a bowl combine almond meal, flour, salt, soda, and baking powder. Pour melted Earth Balance and the rest of the honey into dry mixture; stir until well mixed. Spread evenly over apples. Bake at 350 degrees for 30-45 minutes until bubbly and golden brown.

GINGERBREAD PEOPLE COOKIES

⅔ c. Brown Rice Flour

⅓ c. Sweet Rice Flour

⅓ c. Tapioca Starch Flour

1 T. Cinnamon

1 tsp. Ginger

2 tsp. Xanthan Gum

1 tsp. Baking Soda

½ tsp. Sea Salt

¼ c. Raw Sugar

¼ c. Olive Oil

¼ c. Molasses

2 T. Water

Preheat oven to 350 degrees. Combine dry ingredients in a large bowl. Add oil, molasses, and water. Mix well, adding more tapioca flour as needed to make a soft dough that can be kneaded. Roll out on a tapioca-flour-dusted surface to a thickness of ¼ inch. Cut out with gingerbread people cutters, dipping cutters into tapioca flour after each use. Bake on an ungreased cookie sheet for about 14 minutes. Remove from pan when hot and cool on a wire rack. Cookies will be slightly chewy.

APPLESAUCE CUPCAKES

1 cup Brown Rice Flour

1 cup Millet Flour

1 tsp. Xanthan Gum

1 tsp. Baking Soda

½ tsp. Ground Nutmeg

½ tsp. Ground Cinnamon

¼ tsp. Ground Cloves

¼ tsp. Sea Salt

⅓ c. Earth Balance

¾ cup Honey

1 c. Unsweetened Applesauce

1 c. Raisins (optional)

¼ cup chopped Walnuts
  (optional)

Preheat oven to 350 degrees. Put cupcake liners into cupcake pan. Mix flours, xanthan gum, soda, spices, and salt into a small bowl. Put Earth Balance into mixing bowl and whip until fluffy. Add honey and beat for 2 minutes. Add 1/2 applesauce and 1/2 flour mix to honey/butter mixture. Mix at medium speed until just blended. Add remaining applesauce and flour mixture. Mix again until well blended. Batter will be thick. Stir in raisins and nuts if desired. Spoon batter into cupcake pan. Bake for 25-30 minutes.

◆Great plain or with cream cheese frosting (Page 216).

SMOOTHIE RECIPES

◆*For added immunity boost, add juice from one lemon to any of these.*

DIRECTIONS: To prepare all smoothies, place ingredients into a blender and blend on high until smooth.

THE IMMUNE BOOSTER

1 very ripe Banana

2 handfuls of Frozen Blueberries

1 T. Flaxseed Oil

1 handful Frozen Rasp-
  berries

1 c. Orange Juice or Organic Apple Juice (no sugar)

EVERYTHING SMOOTHIE

1 c. Organic Apple Juice

1 c. Frozen Blueberries

1 Avocado

1 T. Organic Beet Juice (or
  ½ c. Kagome Purple Roots
  and Fruits Juice)

½ c. Carrot Juice

½ c. Frozen Raspberries

2 T. Flaxseed Oil

1 tsp. Juice Organic Lemon
  (or juice from 1 lemon)

FAMILY FAVORITE

1 c. Organic Apple Juice

1 c. Blueberries

1 Carrot

2 Bananas (frozen)

2 handfuls Spinach

Liver Cleanser- bold flavor

1 c. Organic Apple Juice

1 c. Frozen Blueberries

½ c. Frozen Organic Raspberries

2 ripe Bananas

3 T. Organic Beet Juice

FRUITY LIVER REFRESHER

1 c. Organic Apple Juice

1 c. Kagome: Purple Fruits
  & Roots Juice

½ Avocado

3 ripe Bananas

Juice of ½ Organic Lemon
  or 2 T. juiced Lemon

1 c. Frozen Blueberries

LIVER CLEANSER - MILD FLAVOR

1 c. Kagome Purple Roots &
  Fruits Juice

1 c. Organic Apple Juice

1 c. Frozen Blueberries

Juice from 1 Organic Lemon

3 ripe Bananas

SMOOTH-A-LICIOUS!

¼ c. Carrot Juice

2 T. Flaxseed Oil

1 c. Organic Apple Juice

1 very ripe Banana

½ Avocado

1 c. Frozen Organic Blueberries

½ c. Frozen Organic Raspberries (*optional*)

RUBY RED

1 c. Organic Apple Juice

½ Avocado

1 c. Kagome Ruby Red Pomegranate Harmony (or any pomegranate juice)

3 very ripe Bananas

1 c. Blueberries

2 T. Flaxseed Oil

JUST PEACHY

3 very ripe Bananas

1 c. Blueberries

1 c. Kagome Golden Peach Garden (or any peach juice)

½ Avocado

2 T. Flaxseed oil

1 c. Organic Apple Juice

BRAINY POWER FOODS

◆*Low glycemic index foods contribute to MAXIMUM mental performance.*

BRAIN-FRIENDLY PROTEINS

TRYPTOPHAN: comes from the diet and makes serotonin that calms and relaxes the brain.

Foods with tryptophan: 75% dark chocolate, bean items (burritos, rice and bean, etc.), nuts and seeds, legumes.

TYROSINE: not essential because the body can produce it. It makes dopamine, epinephrine, norepinephrine, which rev up the brain.

Foods with Tyrosine: seafood, soy, meat, eggs, and dairy.

Also: avocados (especially overripe), bananas, canned figs (overripe), miso soup, red plums, raisins, sauerkraut*, soy sauce, spinach, teriyaki, tomatoes, beef or chicken liver*, fish, sausages (bologna, pepperoni, salami, summer sausage)*, game meat*, meat tenderizer, meat extracts, caviar, salted herring and other dried fish, pickled herring (spoiled)*, shrimp paste.

*indicates very high levels of Tyrosine

BRAIN-FRIENDLY FATS

◆DHA from cold-water fish is very important for optimal brain functioning.

◆In addition to supplementation sources are: tuna, salmon, flaxseed.

◆Fish and Flax are the TOP BRAIN BUILDING FOODS for growing children.

TIPS

◆Crunchy foods alert the brain and help children to focus: apples, carrots, pears, crackers with soy, rice or goat cheese, chips (occasionally), pickles, and the like.

◆High sugared foods and snacks, especially between meals, are likely to hinder learning and behavior.

◆Fat slows the absorption of sugars. So, if your kids have a high sugar treat, pair it with a good fat such as nuts. (Sugar in ice cream has a lower glycemic index than sugar in frozen yogurt.)

◆Eating low glycemic foods along with highly sugared foods lessens the effects of the fast-acting sugars on the blood sugar.

◆Eating too much at a meal diminishes mental performance.

◆Low calorie + high protein + complex carbs = a brain that is alert and ready to learn.

◆For optimal learning, skip dessert at lunchtime.

THE PERFECT LUNCH

◆High in tyrosine-containing proteins

◆Moderate in the amount of sugars, mainly contain complex carbo-hydrates-low glycemic index

LOW CALORIE GREAT LUNCH IDEAS

◆Salad

◆Black beans, rice, and salsa

◆GF tortillas, goat, rice or soy cheese, black beans, and salsa

◆Tuna subs, sandwiches, melts

◆Pasta with olive oil and pecorino (or nutritional yeast) cheese

◆Goat, rice or soy cheese grilled sandwiches

GRAB & GO SNACKS

Kola Crispy Bars	Larabars
Raisins	Cheddar Bunnies
Blueberries	Dried Blueberries
Dried Cranberries	Dried Apricots – L

Dried Mango

Cashew Packs

PB or Sun Butter Tortillas (Ivory Teff)

Soy Crisps – (limited)

Terra Stix Carrot Packs

Pea Crisps

Sunflower Seeds & Raisins

Macadamia Nuts

Bananas

Pears

Popcorn

Strawberries

Grape Tomatoes

Long Carrots

GF Pretzels

Walnuts

Avocados

Almonds – TJ

Veggie Chips

Crackers or Celery w/Sun Butter or Peanut Butter

Nana's Cookies (GF)

Peapods

Sunflower Seeds

Sunflower Seeds w/Cranberries

Currants

Apples

Peaches

Raspberries

Raw Green Beans

Jerky

Muffins – homemade

Peanuts

Nut Packs

Fruitabu – Fruit Treat

Freeze Dried: Mango Pineapple, Bananas, Strawberries, Rambutan

HEALTHIER CHOICES FOR COMMON ITEMS

BAKING POWDER often has aluminum in it. Aluminum has been linked to Alzheimer's disease and should be *avoided* at all times. Make sure to only use aluminum-free baking powder in your baking.

ALUMINUM FOIL should *NEVER* be used to store or cook food. The use of foil leaches aluminum into your food. Always line the foil with parchment paper before using it. This protects your food from the foil and keeps it free from contamination.

OLIVE OIL should be expeller or cold-pressed to get maximum nutritional value from it.

PURE VANILLA – Make sure the vanilla you use in your baking is pure vanilla that does not contain *vanillin*, a synthetic form of vanilla that is made from by-products of the paper industry. This by-product is added to ethyl vanillin, which is a coal-tar derivative.

ORGANIC KETCHUP contains sugar rather than high fructose corn syrup, so it's the best choice! (Sugar is not "good" for you; however, it's much better for you than HFCG.)

CALCIUM SUPPLEMENTS – When taking a calcium supplement, always take it at bedtime. The magnesium in it will relax your muscles for easy sleeping and your stomach will be empty so there won't be any interference from iron. Iron impedes the absorption of calcium into the body.

SEA SALT – Always use sea salt; it's the least refined and will not affect blood pressure.

GOOD OILS to fry with: expeller or cold pressed olive oil (slowly: low to moderate temperature), and organic coconut oil.

INTERNAL COOKING TEMPERATURE GUIDE

FOR MEAT/LEFTOVERS/CASSEROLES:

(as recommended by the USDA)

◆*Degrees Fahrenheit. The FDA does not recommend Rare 140 degrees as a safe eating temperature.*

Meat	Rare	Med. Rare	Medium	Well Done
Beef	140	145	160	170
Lamb	140	145	160	170
Grnd Beef	-	-	-	160
Veal, Lamb	-	-	-	160
Fresh Pork	-	-	160	170
Fresh Ham	-	-	-	160
Pre-Cooked Ham	-	-	-	140
Chicken/ Turkey (whole)	-	-	-	180
Chicken/ Turkey (ground)	-	-	-	165

Meat	Rare	Med. Rare	Medium	Well Done
Chkn Breast	-	-	-	170
Duck, Goose	-	-	-	180
Leftovers	-	-	-	165
Casseroles	-	-	-	165

RESOURCES

These are doctors that I have consulted with or read their materials in my research. Feel free to contact them or explore their information for more depth in your own personal research. I have also listed the books that I have used in my study of health and nutrition.

Dr. ShaRhae Matousek
Real Health Chiropractic, Eden Prairie, MN
realhealthclinic.com

Dr. Joseph Mercola
mercola.com

Dr. Ben Learner
maximizedlivingdrblerner.com

Dr. Don Colbert
The Seven Pillars of Health, Video Series
drcolbert.com

Dr. Catharine D. Reed
Southlake Pediatrics
southlakepediatrics.com

Anne Packard Spicer, DC
nwhealth.edu/natcare/bios/spicer.html

WEBSITES:

Organic foods and labeling: University of Michigan Health Systems
uofmhealth.org/health-library/

Meat Labels:
suite101.com/content/whats-in-a-meat-label-a22380

Go, Slow, Whoa! A Kid's Guide to Eating Right:
kidshealth.org/kid/nutrition/food/go_slow_whoa.html

Milk, MSG:
Curezone.com/foods/milk.asp *and* curezone.com/foods/msg.asp

Food Colors/Additives:
www.fabresearch.org/789

Food labels:
thechildrenshospital.org/wellness/info/teens/20464.aspx

Organic Foods, Safe Beauty Products, Environmental Workers Group:
foodnews.org

BOOKS

Dr. Don Colbert, *The Seven Pillars of Health,* (Siloam Press , 2007)

Helen Gustafson & Maureen O'Shea, *The Candida Directory and Cookbook,* (Celestial Arts, 1994)

Carol Stock Kranowitz, M.A., *The Out-of-Sync Child: Recognizing and Coping With Sensory Processing Disorder,* revised edition (Perigee, 2005)

James Dobson, *The Strong-Willed Child*, (Tyndale House Publishers, 1985)

Sally Fallon with Mary G. Enig, Ph.D., *Nourishing Traditions*, (Newtrends Publishing, Inc., October 1999)

Dr. Joseph Mercola & Kendra Degen Pearsall, *Sweet Deception*, (Nelson Books, November 2006)

Alternative Medicine: The Definitive Guide, Larry Trivieri, Jr. & John W. Anderson - Editors, Celestial Arts, (June 2002)

Phyllis A. Balch, *Prescription for Nutritional Healing*, 4th edition, (CNC, Avery Trade, October 2006)

From Asparagus to Zucchini: A Guide to Cooking Farm-Fresh Seasonal Produce, 3rd Edition, (Madison Area Community Supported Agriculture Coalition, September 2004)

William G. Crook, *The Yeast Connection: A Medical Breakthrough*, (Vintage Books, September 1986)

Jeanne Lemlin, *Simple Vegetarian Pleasures*, (William Morrow Cookbooks, May 2000)

MOVIE

Foodmatters, Permacology Production (2008), Anto Skene, Director

DIGGING DEEPER

CORN & HFCS & ARTIFICIAL SWEETENERS

King Corn: You Are What You Eat, Documentary, (Mosaic Films, 2007), Aaron Woolf, Director

Joseph Mercola and Kendra Degan Pearsall, *Sweet Deception: Why Splenda, NutraSweet, and the FDA May Be Hazardous to Your Health,* (Nelson Books, 2006)

Sweetpoison, Janet Starr Hull, http//www.sweetpoison.com

Artifiial Sweeteners, Green Facts: Facts on Health and the Environment, http://www.greenfacts.org/en/aspartame/artificial-sweeteners.htm

MSG

If It's Safe: Why Do They Disguise It On The Label?, Sixwise.com, http://shop.sixwise.com/msgifitssafewhydotheydisguiseitonlabels42605.aspx (4/26/05)

MSGTruth.org, http://www.msgtruth.org/

FOOD COLORING

Ben F. Fiengold, M.D, *Why Your Child Is Hyperactive* (Random House, 1985)

Feingold Association of theUnited States, http://www.feingold.org/

Chemical Cuisine: Learn About Food Additives, Center for Science in the Public Interest, http://www.cspinet.org/reports/chemcuisine.htm

Good Fats

Fallon and Enig, *Nourishing Traditions: The Cookbook that Challenges Politically Correct Nutrition and the Diet Dictocrats*, (New Trends Publishing, 2001)

7 Reasons to Eat More Saturated Fat, Mercola.com: Take Control of Your Health, http://articles.mercola.com/sites/articles/archive/2009/09/22/7-Reasons-to-Eat-More-Saturated-Fat.aspx

Dr. Joseph Mercola, *Coconut Oil Benefits: When Fat is Good for You*, The Huffington Post, February 14, 2011, http://www.huffingtonpost.com/dr-mercola/coconut-oil-benefits_b_821453.html

Vin Miller, *12 Reasons Why Saturated Fat is Good For You*, Natural Bias: Maximizing Life Through Health, Fitness and Perspective, naturalbias.com/12-reasons-why-saturated-fat-is-good-for-you (October 16th, 2009)

Healthy Meat

Jo Johnson, *Why Grassfed is Best!*, American Grass Fed Beef.com, The Health Benefits of Grass Farming, http://www.americangrassfedbeef.com/grass-fed-natural-beef.asp

Eatwild: The #1 Site for Grass-fed food and facts, http://www.eatwild.com/

Dairy

Dave Rietz, *Dangers of Milk and Dairy Products, The Facts*, http://www.rense.com/general26/milk.htm

Robert Cohen, *Milk A-Z*, (Argus Publishing, 2001)

Pure Water

Safe Drinking Water Act, EPA: United States Environmental Protection Agency, http://water.epa.gov/lawsregs/rulesregs/sdwa/

Bottled Water Quality Investigation: 10 Major Brands, 38 Pollutants, Environmental Working Group, http://www.ewg.org/reports/Bottled Water/Bottled-Water-Quality-Investigation

Water, The Miracle Cure, Divine Health, Dr. Don Colbert M.D., http://www.drcolbert.com/cont_articles.php?view=full&artcat =2&aid=132

The Most Important Nutrient in the Body, Divine Health, Dr. Don Colbert M.D., http://www.drcolbert.com/cont_articles. php?view=full&artcat=3&aid=49

Whole Grains

The Dr.com, http://www.thedr.com/

Living Without: The Magazine for People with Alergies and Food Sensitivities, http://www.livingwithout.com/

Celiac.com, Celiac Disease and Gluten-free Diet Information Since 1995, http://www.celiac.com/

Labels

So What Exactly Does "Certified Organic" Mean? Is It Really Organic?, www.sixwise.com, (Newsletter 5/12/07)

Food Nutrition Labels: Six Catches You Need To Know. www.sixwise. com, (Newsletter 5/11/02)

BRANDS

The Sneaky Chef

Nature's Path

Bob's Red Mill

Bob's Red Mill Wonderful
  Bread Mix

Drew's

Fruitabu

Tofutti

Glutino's

So Delicious

Kagome Fruit Juices

Larabar

Nordic Naturals (known for
  their high quality and purity)

Kinnikinnick Foods

Van's Natural Foods

Bob's Red Mill Biscuit Mix

Earth Balance

Enrico's

Spectrum

Apple Gate Farms

Mini Belle

Zevia

Kola

Terra Stix

SunSpire (Truly Inspired
  Natural Chocolate) for
  SunDrops